Technological Advances in Care of Patients with Kidney Diseases

Subodh J. Saggi • Moro O. Salifu
Editors

Technological Advances in Care of Patients with Kidney Diseases

Springer

Editors
Subodh J. Saggi
Medicine
SUNY Downstate Medical Center
Brooklyn, NY, USA

Moro O. Salifu
Medicine
SUNY Downstate Medical Center
Brooklyn, NY, USA

ISBN 978-3-031-11941-5 ISBN 978-3-031-11942-2 (eBook)
https://doi.org/10.1007/978-3-031-11942-2

This Springer imprint is published by the registered company Springer Nature Switzerland AG
The registered company address is: Gewerbestrasse 11, 6330 Cham, Switzerland

Preface

About 10 years ago we began a series of symposiums yearly at SUNY Downstate Health Sciences University, Brooklyn, New York, to recognize the advances being made in the realm of kidney diseases, both preventative and therapeutic. Most providers that take care of patients with kidney diseases are usually engrossed in the day-to-day care of patients on renal replacement therapies such as dialysis. Providers who live their life taking care of such patients learn rather quickly their patient's grief, their pain, and a yearning for freedom from their daily grind of doing dialysis to survive. It is truly tiring and exhaustive. Every day they see the same providers, the same nursing staff, the same housekeeper, and the same front desk staff. Such staff become their family over time. There is no family that does not have internal squabbles or friction, but in the end being family everything is forgiven and forgotten.

Somewhere along this journey of our patients and providers someone begins to listen to our patients cries and notices their tears. Hope begins to take seed and provide them the freedom they yearn for with the arrival of a kidney from an altruistic donor. It is said that freedom is earned and not given. Thus, when providers and patients both try their utmost best to hold on to their faith something wonderful happens that day. Transplantation is a true miracle of science just as dialysis was. We cannot but think and pause to recognize the many decades of struggles of so many scientists, researchers, patients, and philanthropists who themselves fought so many odds to continue their journey of supporting and providing that hope to our patients.

How does this first edition of this book do any justice to our patients, dialysis workforce, or transplant workforce? In our planning of the first symposium which we designed and then designed every year for the past decade, we wanted to recognize and thank the bond that exists between patients and providers. We learn from our patients, and until providers are patients themselves their grief is not truly sensed. We thought very carefully as to what gets lost during their journey for providers and patients on dialysis? No one can replace lost time but what we thought we could give them instead is a memoir of the achievements and work still being done in kidney diseases. We wanted to let them know that we as doctors are still listening to their fears, we are not numb. This book is thus a dedication to the efforts of so many scientists that are eager to share and reflect on their achievements. Each milestone each year is a journey of their struggles. We were asked by many who wrote such wonderful chapters in this book whether this book is for the providers or for the patients? For a moment we hesitated in answering because deep down we wondered whether such a question was even appropriate because in the end unless a provider is a patient themselves how in the world will they truly understand the grief? A true scientific investigative journey does not begin with a wrong hypothesis. How can we as providers begin to hypothesize and find cures if we do not know what troubles our patients when their kidneys fail or when they go on dialysis or when their transplanted kidney begins to fail yet once again?

We have laid out in this book work being done in identifying root causes of kidney failure such as aberrant gene expressions or when investigation into genetic causes is required, or when investigation into abnormal metabolism or the collected accumulation of abnormal metabolites causes organ dysfunction, among an array of reasons why kidneys faulter. We have delved further into how our environment particularly our nutrition plays an integral part in generating abnormal metabolites that are toxic and add further insult to the failing kidney and other organs and what can we do to prevent it? More importantly what can our patients do, how can they access appropriate resources of healthy nutrition? Can nutrition be therapeutic?

There is no article one can pick up today which does not mention the bulk of kidney diseases result from diabetes and hypertension. We asked our colleagues to write about, not only what is known about diabetes when it affects the kidney but to write about how our patients can manage the two diseases together and what evidence exists as to what really works. We thus invited some colleagues to write about how best to harness the power of technology in the space of kidney diseases. As many interventional experiments cannot be performed without ethical inquiry, rigorous statistical methodical approaches of observational and retrospective large data analysis fill the gap. We call this artificial intelligence, a term that creates fear in many, both patients and providers. But what we have personally learned from this journey is that it does provide tremendous insight and helps steer us in the right direction for better ideas on how to provide and receive care.

Technology has had a major impact in the way we manage our patients with kidney disease both on dialysis within a hemodialysis center or at home. The COVID 19 pandemic showed us how much infection control plays a role in managing the life of a patient on dialysis. Simple tasks such as proper hand washing and careful vigilance to every step in starting a patient on a treatment to terminating their treatment have had a complex array of steps that seemed superficial some time ago but now is rooted in better outcomes. Technology has provided us this insight. Remote monitoring of patients on home dialysis seemed like science fiction at one point which is now the norm. We asked one of my close colleagues to write about such advancements for our patients to read and understand how being on home dialysis lets them do dialysis safely in the comfort of their home and loved ones while we as providers could manage and monitor them safely. Here once again we see our bond between us as providers and our patients.

Cardiac disease affects all our patients with kidney diseases and by the time they land on dialysis their vascular system is damaged. Noninvasive placement of vascular access is emerging as an alternative to surgical placement in qualified patients. One chapter is dedicated to noninvasive vascular access creation.

We thank all the authors who have spent enormous amounts of time developing these chapters. We dedicate this first edition to all patients with kidney failure and to our eminent mentor Dr. Eli A. Friedman, Distinguished Teaching Professor Emeritus and founder of the nephrology division at SUNY Downstate and subsequently performing the first federally funded hemodialysis in the United States in 1963.

Brooklyn, NY, USA Subodh J. Saggi
Brooklyn, NY, USA Moro O. Salifu

Contents

Chapter 1
Genetic Testing for the Management of Kidney Disease

Sindhuri Prakash and Jordan G. Nestor

Individuals with advanced kidney disease represent a growing population in the USA and the world, contributing to significant morbidity, mortality, and healthcare expenditure. Worldwide increase in kidney disease prevalence is attributed to an aging population and the co-incident increase in diabetes and hypertension [1, 2]. In the USA, the prevalence of kidney disease is estimated to be 15% of the population, roughly accounting for over 30 million Americans and sadly, the incidence of kidney failure is projected to increase by 11–13% by 2030 [3].

Despite efforts to capture patients in the early stages of kidney disease, many patients present late to nephrology care, illustrated by the fact that a third of incident kidney failure patients had no pre-nephrology care in 2017 [2]. This is largely due to the asymptomatic nature of disease in its nascent stages, as many patients are unaware of developing kidney disease until they have progressed to renal failure. Moreover, fewer than 10% of patients with kidney disease are aware of the impact of kidney health and mortality [4], representing a paucity in patient education. This leads to challenges in diagnosis and treatment, as patients need renal replacement therapy promptly in a time sensitive manner and cannot afford to have a management plan focused on mitigating progression of kidney failure. They also present with diagnostic challenges, as they are typically precluded from a biopsy, as kidney failure is characterized by high degree of interstitial fibrosis and an underlying diagnosis cannot be observed. Although a large portion of patients have comorbid conditions such as diabetes and hypertension, which comprise 60% of cases of kidney failure, patients with progressive kidney dysfunction develop hypertension as a complication. While this may or may not be the primary driver of organ failure in these patients, patients are given the putative diagnosis of hypertension as their underlying etiology of kidney failure. Moreover, in many instances, once a patient

S. Prakash · J. G. Nestor (✉)
Department of Medicine, Division of Nephrology, Columbia University, New York, NY, USA
e-mail: sp2518@cumc.columbia.edu; jgn2108@cumc.columbia.edu

S. J. Saggi, M. O. Salifu (eds.), *Technological Advances in Care of Patients with Kidney Diseases*, https://doi.org/10.1007/978-3-031-11942-2_1

is diagnosed with advanced kidney disease, it may not be readily apparent that a search for an etiology of kidney disease will change management, impact transplantation or affect family planning.

Interestingly, kidney function and kidney disease often are heritable [5, 6], with 25% of patients reporting it in their family history [7, 8]. In addition, 10% of kidney disease cases are thought to be Mendelian in nature [9]. Registries from both the USA and Europe report 15–20% of patients with kidney failure of unknown etiology [2, 10] and studies conducted thus far report a genetic diagnosis in 17–38% of this subset of patients [8, 11]. Traditionally, determining the etiology of an individual's nephropathy involves taking a comprehensive medical and family history, and review of biochemical assays, imaging studies, and histopathology. However, there is substantial overlap in clinical presentation and histopathology of both acquired and hereditary forms of kidney disease, which makes it difficult to distinguish the two using traditional diagnostic tools. To combat this, clinical genetic testing, including genome-wide approaches such exome and genome sequencing, are increasingly being used in the clinical setting, including in nephrology [12, 13]. In one study, among patients who underwent genetic testing, 40% had confirmation of their suspected diagnosis while 22% underwent correction or reclassification of their clinical diagnosis [14]. Establishing a diagnosis in these patients can have many benefits, which include early diagnosis, prognostication, personalized care, guide decisions on transplantation, and allow family planning [15]. This chapter will focus on how the use of genetic tests can shape diagnosis and management in advanced kidney disease, select patients at who are at risk for rapid progression, and impact transplantation and renal replacement therapies. This chapter will also serve to provide a brief compendium on the types of genetic modalities available, when to refer patients to genetics, and how genetics can inform ongoing care for patients with kidney disease.

Rationale for the Use of Genetic Tests in Diagnosing Kidney Disease

Inherited susceptibility to kidney dysfunction can either be due to a variation in a single gene (monogenic) that has a large effect on kidney function, called a Mendelian disorder, or due to the cumulative effect of variation in many genes that contribute to disease development (complex genetic disease). The number of genes implicated in kidney function and disease has expanded tremendously in the last decade and will continue to increase over time. As more data continue to be gathered for kidney phenotypes with genomic sequencing, and cell specific expression profiles are being generated in various kidney diseases, the list of potential genes involved in kidney disease will exponentially increase over the coming decades. Thus, sequencing for genes associated with kidney diseases should be part of the diagnostic armamentarium for patients with kidney disease.

Although Mendelian forms of kidney disease are traditionally thought be enriched in pediatric cases, up to 40% of adults with kidney disease who have a positive family history, have a monogenic form of kidney disease [13, 14]. These studies demonstrate that overall diagnostic rates of a monogenic cause of kidney disease between adults and children are not statistically different when clinicians have a high suspicion of an inherited kidney disease. Albeit, some diseases are more prevalent in their expected age groups, for example, children had higher prevalence of congenital anomalies of the kidney and urologic tract (CAKUT) and adults had higher diagnoses of Alport syndrome, but the overall diagnostic outcome with genetic modalities is not affected by age [13]. Similar to monogenic diseases in pediatrics, patients with a positive family history who present at a younger age and exhibit extra-renal features represent a patient population that should be selected for genetic testing as they are more likely to have an inherited form of kidney disease. Thus, a comprehensive family history should be taken for all patients in a nephrology clinic. In addition, patients categorized as having kidney disease of unknown etiology represent another population where patients have a higher likelihood of having a hereditary cause [14]. As proof of principle, among patients who underwent genetic testing with a positive return of diagnosis, 36% had family history of kidney disease, and 69% had extra-renal manifestations [14]. More importantly, there was no difference in the median age group between patients with a genetic diagnosis and those without. Interestingly, among patients who carried the diagnosis of kidney disease of unknown etiology, 47% were found to have a monogenic cause, and 15% of patients did not have family history or extra-renal manifestations, pointing to the utility of genetics in kidney disease, diagnosis irrespective of the cardinal features of monogenic disease [14]. Similarly, many diseases that are traditionally thought to be pediatric may be under-diagnosed in adulthood, such as in nephronophthisis, a common cause of kidney failure in children. Variants in *NPHP1* are now known to be a frequent cause of adult onset kidney failure, where more than 50% of patients present after age 30, and a large portion of patients were classified as having kidney disease unknown [16].

Establishing Genetic Diagnoses Impacts Clinical Care

The most common monogenic kidney disease is autosomal dominant polycystic kidney disease (ADPKD), caused by mutations in *PKD1* and *PKD2*. Traditionally, patients are diagnosed based on family history, early onset of hypertension and ultrasound criteria of a higher kidney volume to height ratio. The clinical presentation of ADPKD is varied with patients presenting with hypertension, hematuria, proteinuria or kidney failure. Patients with mutations in *PKD1* have a worse prognosis with earlier onset of kidney failure. Moreover patients with milder clinical course are more likely to harbor non-truncating mutations such as single nucleotide polymorphisms called missense mutations, which might be missed using clinical criteria alone [17]. Moreover imaging does not distinguish between other acquired cystic diseases (such as advanced kidney disease or renal cell carcinoma), and other hereditary forms of cystic diseases, including autosomal dominant tubulointerstitial disease (ADTKD), which can cause kidney failure without kidney enlargement, or autosomal recessive polycystic kidney disease (ARPKD), which causes fibrosis. In addition, mutations in *GANAB* or *DNAJB11* cause a mild form of cystic disease that may not progress to kidney failure. Patients with ADPKD also have lesions in their liver and brain, and patients who are undetected are at risk for death from sudden intracranial aneurysmal rupture. Having a genetic diagnosis therefore is definitive and not just presumptive and will be helpful for many reasons. These include prognostication of patients who are at risk for kidney failure and counseling of close relatives. Also, it allows clinicians to identify patients who are candidates for tolvaptan therapy, a V2 receptor antagonist that inhibits cyst formation [18]. Currently patients are selected based on age, kidney size length, rate of decline in eGFR and the Mayo classification for tolvaptan therapy [19]. Genetic diagnosis can allow clinicians to select these patients in the pre-symptomatic stage for early treatment, before patients develop liver function test abnormalities, which precludes them from tolvaptan treatment. Patients who are diagnosed with ADPKD in child bearing age can also participate in assisted reproductive strategies to reduce the risk of passing on the mutation to future generations [20].

Alport syndrome is an inherited hematuric glomerulopathy characterized by progressive kidney dysfunction, hearing loss and ocular abnormalities. Alport syndrome occurs due to mutations in any of the three type IV collagen genes *COL4A3/4/5*, which encode the triple helix of the glomerular basement membranes, cochlea and various components of the eye including the retina, lens capsule and cornea. Inheritance is X-linked in the majority of cases (85%), though there are also autosomal forms of inheritance. Penetrance can be variable as disease severity varies within Alport spectrum phenotypes, ranging from microscopic hematuria with stable kidney function, to early onset kidney failure with auditory and visual impairments, and even isolated focal segmental glomerulosclerosis (FSGS) pattern lesions [21, 22]. Similar to ADPKD, the type of genetic mutation may also modulate disease severity, with individuals with missense variants displaying milder disease (e.g., hematuria and proteinuria with less severe audiologic and ocular involvement) versus those with loss-of-function mutations (e.g., nonsense, frameshift or deletions) who develop kidney failure [23–25]. However, in Alport syndrome, a missense variant at a glycine residue of the collagen triple helix molecule with a charged residue can also result in a more severe phenotype [26]. Males with X-linked Alport syndrome (due to a mutation in *COL4A5*) have a greater risk for kidney failure between the second and sixth decades of life, develop hearing loss and ocular changes. As obligate heterozygotes, females generally show a milder disease course, however, studies have shown that approximately 15–30% go on to develop kidney failure, and almost a third developed sensorineural hearing loss [23, 24, 27]. Kidney biopsy can be avoided if a molecular diagnosis is established through genetic testing, which is more sensitive and specific for the diagnosis of Alport syndrome [28]. Individuals with Alport syndrome should be referred for audiometry, ophthalmologic review, including retinal imaging and retinal optical coherence tomography if possible [29, 30]. In addition, the patients should have close monitoring of kidney function and blood pressure treatment with RAAS blockade such as an ACE-inhibitor to ameliorate proteinuria and progression of kidney failure [29, 31] Patients should be referred to transplantation early. Though patients generally have positive outcomes after transplantation, but a rare and devastating consequence in the post-transplant period is anti-GBM nephritis as patients are immunologically naïve and form antibodies against the donor GBM proteins. This occurs in patients mostly with X-linked Alport syndrome who have truncating mutations 2–3% of the time [32]. Donor selection is complex in Alport syndrome as many family members can have differing risks for kidney failure based on their genotype. For example, women with X-linked Alport syndrome can frequently develop kidney disease, and often will preclude them from being candidate donors to affected family members [33]. Heterozygote mutations in *COL4A3 and COL4A5* can have variable presentation, and donor candidacy may vary depending on the presence or absence of the phenotype.

Establishing the genetic underpinning of patients with albuminuria or FSGS pattern lesions who are suspected of having a monogenic disease is very important for personalization of their care [34, 35]. Though not a stand-alone clinical diagnosis, FSGS has historically been divided in two main forms: primary and secondary [36]. Today, there are increasing opportunities to further distinguish the genetic forms of disease, which are caused by mutations in various proteins, including those that form the podocyte slit diaphragm, the glomerular basement membrane, mitochondria, lysosome and the cytoskeletal and nuclear compartments (see Table 1.1). Unlike primary FSGS, which is thought to be caused by a circulating factor and often treated with corticosteroids and immunomodulatory agents, genetic forms of FSGS can have variable steroid response rates [38]. Therefore, diagnostic findings for a genetic form of FSGS may guide clinicians away from prescribing corticosteroids [39], sparing the patient of unwanted side effects such as weight gain, hyperglycemia, and bone loss. The diagnosis may instead steer them toward more aggressive blood pressure management, using agents that inhibit the RAAS pathway, in an effort to decrease the amount of proteinuria and potentially slow the rate of disease progression. The genetic diagnosis may also provide prognostic insights, as hereditary forms are associated with lower recurrence rate after kidney transplantation [40]. Genetic testing can also help identify cases that may benefit from targeted therapies, as in case of mutations in genes of the CoQ10 biosynthesis pathway (i.e., *ADCK4*, *COQ2*, *COQ6*, or *PDSS2*) that respond to CoQ10 supplementation [41–44], and alert clinicians and patients to ongoing clinical trials [45]. To date, more than 50 genes have been implicated with genetic forms of FSGS (Table 1.1) [46, 47]. The pace of discovery for new gene associated with this clinical entity is rapidly growing due to the more extensive use of genetic testing in clinical care. Furthermore, different genes are related to different clinical manifestations with varying age of onset, that can be either kidney-limited or part of a multiorgan syndrome [46, 48].

Variants in *APOL1* that protect against African sleeping sickness caused by trypanosomes are associated with increased risk of kidney disease. Having two copies

Table 1.1 Examples of major genes associated with genetic forms of FSGS (adapted from Clinical Genetic Screening in adult patients with kidney disease, CJASN) [37]

Protein	Gene	Inheritance	Location	Function of the encoded protein
Slit diaphragm proteins				
Nephrin	*NPHS1*	AR	19q13.1	Member of the immunoglobulin family, cell adhesion molecules
Podocin	*NPHS2*	AR	1q25 31	Regulation of glomerular permeability
CD2 associated protein	*CD2AP*	AD (AR)	6p12	Scaffolding molecule that regulates the actin cytoskeleton
Cell membrane associated proteins				
Transient receptor potential cation channel 6	*TRPC6*	AD	11q21 22	Receptor-activated calcium channel in the cell membrane
Protein tyrosine phosphatase receptor type O	*PTPRO*	AR	12p22	Member of the R3 subtype family of protein tyrosine phosphatases at the apical surface of polarized cells
Laminin 2	*LAMB2*	AR	3p21	Family of extracellular matrix glycoproteins in the basement membranes
4 integrin	*ITGB4*	AR	17q11	Transmembrane glycoprotein receptors
Tetraspanin CD151	*CD151*	AR	11p15	Member of the transmembrane 4 superfamily, cell-surface proteins
LIM homeobox transcription factor 1β	*LMX1B*	AD	9q33.3	Member of LIM-homeodomain family, transcription factor
Cytosolic or cytoskeletal proteins				
Actinin 4	*ACTN4*	AD	19q13	Member of the spectrin gene superfamily, cytoskeletal proteins
Phospholipase C1	*PLCE1*	AR	10q23 24	Member of the apolipoprotein C1 family, role in HDL and VLDL metabolism
Myosin heavy chain 9	*MYH9*	AD	22q12.3	Nonmuscle myosin, involved in cytokinesis, cell motility, and maintenance of cell shape
Inverted formin 2	*INF2*	AD	14q32	Member of the formin family, function in de- and polymerization of actin filaments
Myosin 1E	*MYO1E*	AR	15q21 26	Member of the nonmuscle class I myosins, involved in intracellular movement and membrane trafficking

Table 1.1 (continued)

Protein	Gene	Inheritance	Location	Function of the encoded protein
Rho GDP-dissociation inhibitor 1	*ARHGDIA*	AR	17q25	Key role in the regulation of signaling through Rho GTPases
Nuclear proteins				
Wilms tumor 1	*WT1*	AD	11p13	Transcription factor, role in the normal development of the urogenital system
SMARCA-like protein	*SMARCAL1*	AR	2q34 36	Member of the SWI/SNF family, transcription factor
Mitochondrial components				
Para-hydroxybenzoate polyprenyltransferase	*COQ2*	AR	4q21 22	Functions in the final steps in the biosynthesis of CoQ
Coenzyme Q10 biosynthesis monooxygenase 6	*COQ6*	AR	14q24.3	Member of the ubiH/COQ6 family, required for the biosynthesis of coenzyme Q10
Decaprenyl diphosphate synthase subunit 2	*PDSS2*	AR	6q21	Enzyme that synthesizes the prenyl side chain of coenzyme Q or ubiquinone
AarF domain-containing protein kinase 4	*ADCK4*	AR	19q13.2	Precise function unknown (possible protein kinase activity)
Lysosomal proteins				
Lysosomal integral membrane protein type 2	*SCARB2*	AR	4q13 21	Type III glycoprotein located in limiting membranes of lysosomes and endosomes
Unknown cellular location				
Apolipoprotein L1	*APOL1*	AR	22q12	Secreted high-density lipoprotein, involved in the formation of cholesteryl esters and efflux of cholesterol from cells
Glomerular basement membrane				
Collagen type IV alpha 3	*COL4A3*	AR, AD	2q36.3	Major structural component of basement membranes
Collagen type IV alpha 4	*COL4A4*	AR, AD	2q36.3	Major structural component of basement membranes
Collagen type IV alpha 5	*COL4A5*	XLD	Xq22.3	Major structural component of basement membranes

of the risk variants of *APOL1*, known as G1 and G2, increase the risk of kidney failure due to hypertension [49], sickle cell nephropathy [50], progressive lupus [51], HIV associated nephropathy [52], and other viral nephropathies such as COVID-19 [53, 54]. The mechanism by which *APOL1* causes kidney injury is still being worked out, but might be involved in podocyte dysfunction. Nonetheless, patients and donors with *APOL1* high-risk variants have implications for transplantation. Interestingly, donor kidneys with high-risk *APOL1* genotype is seen to contribute to decreased graft function, onset of proteinuria and FSGS, and early graft failure. In addition, donors of high-risk *APOL1* variants develop kidney failure after donation at higher rates [55]. Outcomes data on transplantation of *APOL1* high-risk donors to recipients and underlying etiology of graft failure is still being studied in the APOLLO study. Though the medical actionability of *APOL1* risk variants is still debated, knowing the risk variants in *APOL1* can identify potential living donors who may be at increased risk for *APOL1*-associated nephropathy following donor nephrectomy [56]. In the meantime, in an effort to improve outcomes of transplantation, family members of patients with high-risk *APOL1* genotype who wish to be potential donors should be offered *APOL1* genotyping and counseling regarding the projected implications for their health. While it conceptually warrants genotyping of deceased donor kidneys, ethical implications of such measures must be considered carefully.

Genetic Testing Available in the Clinic

While the hope is to someday perform genetic testing in an unbiased manner, currently genetic testing is not routinely performed for all comers and is undertaken for a select number of patients in conjunction with laboratories equipped with interpretation expertise. Genetic testing can be performed through several different modalities and are chosen to support a clinical diagnosis or when the clinical diagnosis is ambiguous. Therefore, knowledge of the type of tests available and when to use them can be helpful when considering the type of genetic test to offer patients in nephrology clinic. When a patient has a high suspicion of an inherited disorder caused by a specific gene, such as ADPKD, or when confirmation of particular variant is needed in patients or at-risk relatives, Sanger sequencing is the test of choice. This is because Sanger sequencing has high sensitivity and specificity with 99.999% accuracy for each base pair sequenced [57]. The technique is ideal for sequencing short segments that are up to 1000 base pairs long and segments of the genome with repetitive sequences that have a high melting point leading to high chance of error. Patients who have a clinical presentation diagnostic of conditions that are caused by a handful of genes such as nephrotic syndrome, cystic diseases, glomerular diseases or tubulopathies, targeted gene panels can be useful [58, 59]. Patients who present with a syndromic presentation with multiorgan involvement should be tested on a microarray or exome sequencing to pick up chromosomal abnormalities to explain their disease. When patients present with symptoms that are diagnostically ambiguous, and when disease is caused by a multiple genes (genetically heterogeneous) whole exome or genome sequencing is the preferred testing modality. In general, the known clinical and genetic heterogeneity of monogenic nephropathies supports use of exome sequencing as a first-line diagnostic tool for non-cystic kidney diseases [60, 61]. Recent studies show that exome sequencing can pinpoint a hereditary cause in 10–35% of kidney disease patients, including in almost a third of FSGS cases patients [14, 60, 62–70].

Sequence interpretation is extremely important as the goal of genetic testing is to discover a genetic variant that is responsible for the patient's condition. This requires a high degree of accuracy as clinical management decisions are made based on these diagnoses. Genetic analysis is typically time consuming and cumbersome, and a diagnosis should be made in collaboration with experienced geneticists. The clinical presentation is pivotal in guiding variant association to disease. Interpretation of variants can be challenging, where certain mutations can cause a different disease than the one classically implicated for a gene, for example, p.R76W mutation in *HNF4A* causes Fanconi syndrome, while the gene is associated with MODY1 (maturity onset diabetes of the young type 1) [71].

Genomic Approaches and Return of Results

Genome-wide sequencing techniques (i.e., exome and genome sequencing) have greater analytic sensitivity than targeted sequencing approach (e.g., Sanger sequencing, targeted gene panel, etc.), and have the power to return variants that were not expected at the time of testing. These include variants in genes that are diagnostic for monogenic disease or variants in any of the 59 genes that deemed to be medically actionable. Many genes on this list may warrant further nephrology care, such as Fabry's disease, Wilms tumor, hereditary pheochromocytoma-paraganglioma syndrome and Von-Hippau Lindau and tuberous sclerosis. In addition, knowledge of these actionable genes can help provide comprehensive care, such as reducing immunosuppression in transplant patients harboring the *BRCA1* gene or defibrillator implantation in patients with Long QT syndrome or arrhythmogenic right ventricular cardiomyopathy, and increase malignancy screening in patients with Lynch, Peutz-Jeghers or Li-Fraumeni syndromes. These findings are reportable as patients can benefit from a medical intervention. In addition, these approaches also inadvertently provide a clinician with the patient's pharmacogenomic profile that can inform drug dosing and predict adverse drug reactions, such *CYP3A5* expressors who need increasing dosing of tacrolimus for optimal immunosuppression during transplantation [72].

Moreover, these broad genomic approaches increase the chance of identifying variants of unknown significance in protein coding regions or variants in noncoding regions of the genome. These variants are difficult to interpret and assess disease risk for patients. This is similar to receiving incidental findings with imaging that encompasses the entire body in certain clinical scenarios. While they are challenging to interpret during the time of testing, these variants can become clinically relevant as new genetic knowledge is amassed, and variants that were deemed diagnostic can become irrelevant. This factor has huge implications for the patient as these genetic diagnoses impact clinical care. This requires clinicians and genetic laboratories to conduct periodic re-analyses of current data, and current protocols do not delineate time intervals of re-analyses, or which party is responsible for requesting the data. In addition, psychosocial implications should be considered when returning the results of re-analyses to patients and families, especially when a variant is reclassified as pathogenic while it was considered to be otherwise at the time of testing.

Ethical, Legal, Social Considerations and Return of Results

Altogether, returning results of genomic testing to patients carries unique ethical, legal, and social implications that underscore the need for informed consent and comprehensive genetic counseling before sequencing is carried out. Currently, comprehensive pretest counseling is required which addresses the aforementioned issues including expected results of the genetic test including secondary findings, which requires expertise in interpretation of genetic results. Genetic counselors can be incorporated into the clinical care team for the patient, which can aid in result interpretation. If this cannot be accomplished to resource availability, referral to genetics clinic should be done, or tele-health visits with regional experts can be arranged.

It is important to counsel patients and families that genetic testing is a gateway for patients to participate in research. Patients can benefit from being part of research as they can be recruited into clinical trials that impact care, for example in hereditary nephropathies. In addition, genetic data can also contribute to research in identifying new variants or reclassification of variants. In addition, sequencing of minority patients help contribute to the fund of sequence data that allows geneticists to glean a more accurate allele frequency of variants that can prevent over-diagnoses/misdiagnosis of pathogenic variants. This is because variants that are expected to be pathogenic are often rare and sequence data is typically compared to European reference data. As more populations are sequenced, minority specific reference data can be established ameliorating this issue and allowing more accurate diagnosis.

While patients may be hesitant to participate in genetic testing for various reasons, it should be conveyed that genetic information is protected against discrimination under International (under UNESCO), European, and United States law. The genetic information nondiscrimination act forbids employers from having access to genetic information, which would allow them to discriminate against these individuals. However, this does not extend to disability or life insurance, which can dissuade patients from participating in genetic testing.

Summary

Nephrogenomics is an emerging field, where genomics can aid in early diagnosis and management of many patients with kidney failure. Genetic sequencing technologies include many modalities that allow accurate diagnosis of monogenic diseases and chromosomal abnormalities and have the power to detect secondary findings that can be clinically relevant to the patient. Importantly, it allows the diagnosis of patients who are deemed to have unknown etiology and allow accurate diagnosis when the clinical picture is ambiguous. A genetic diagnosis can guide management, including choice of therapy and subspecialty referrals, inform prognosis, and family counseling. Genetic testing can also further research that also allow the creation of a compendium of genes and variants that cause certain diseases and allow better stratification of phenotypes for clinical studies than just relying on clinical parameters alone. More importantly, genetic data allow for personalized care for each patient, as clinical data and genetic risk can inform clinical care for the disease at hand, but also inform future risk for patients and families.

Acknowledgements The project was supported by grants from the National Institutes of Health through grant KL2TR001874 and the National Kidney Foundation's Young Investigator Award (J.G.N.).

Disclosures None.

References

1. Bikbov B, Purcell CA, Levey AS, Smith M, Abdoli A, Abebe M, Adebayo OM, Afarideh M, Agarwal SK, Agudelo-Botero M. Global, regional, and national burden of chronic kidney disease, 1990–2017: a systematic analysis for the Global Burden of Disease Study 2017. Lancet. 2020;395:709–33.
2. Saran R, Robinson B, Abbott KC, Bragg-Gresham J, Chen X, Gipson D, Gu H, Hirth RA, Hutton D, Jin Y. US renal data system 2019 annual data report: epidemiology of kidney disease in the United States. Am J Kidney Dis. 2020;75(1):A6–7.
3. McCullough KP, Morgenstern H, Saran R, Herman WH, Robinson BM. Projecting ESRD incidence and prevalence in the United States through 2030. J Am Soc Nephrol. 2019;30:127–35.
4. Whaley-Connell A, Shlipak MG, Inker LA, Tamura MK, Bomback AS, Saab G, Szpunar SM, McFarlane SI, Li S, Chen S-C. Awareness of kidney disease and relationship to end-stage renal disease and mortality. Am J Med. 2012;125:661–9.
5. Satko SG, Sedor JR, Iyengar SK, Freedman BI. Familial clustering of chronic kidney disease. Semin Dial. 2007;20:229–36.
6. Bello AK, Peters J, Wight J, de Zeeuw D, El Nahas M. A population-based screening for microalbuminuria among relatives of CKD patients: the kidney evaluation and awareness program in Sheffield (KEAPS). Am J Kidney Dis. 2008;52:434–43.
7. McClellan WM, Satko SG, Gladstone E, Krisher JO, Narva AS, Freedman BI. Individuals with a family history of ESRD are a high-risk population for CKD: implications for targeted surveillance and intervention activities. Am J Kidney Dis. 2009;53:S100–6.

8. Connaughton DM, Bukhari S, Conlon P, Cassidy E, O'Toole M, Mohamad M, Flanagan J, Butler T, O'Leary A, Wong L. The irish kidney gene project-prevalence of family history in patients with kidney disease in Ireland. Nephron. 2015;130:293–301.
9. Wühl E, van Stralen KJ, Wanner C, Ariceta G, Heaf JG, Bjerre AK, Palsson R, Duneau G, Hoitsma AJ, Ravani P. Renal replacement therapy for rare diseases affecting the kidney: an analysis of the ERA–EDTA Registry. Nephrol Dial Transplant. 2014;29:1–8.
10. ERA-EDTA Registry. ERA-EDTA registry annual report 2016. Amsterdam: Amsterdam UMC; 2018.
11. Groopman EE, Marasa M, Cameron-Christie S, Petrovski S, Aggarwal VS, Milo-Rasouly H, Li Y, Zhang J, Nestor J, Krithivasan P, et al. Diagnostic utility of exome sequencing for kidney disease. N Engl J Med. 2018;380:142–51.
12. Santin S, Bullich G, Tazon-Vega B, Garcia-Maset R, Gimenez I, Silva I, Ruiz P, Ballarin J, Torra R, Ars E. Clinical utility of genetic testing in children and adults with steroid-resistant nephrotic syndrome. Clin J Am Soc Nephrol. 2011;6:1139–48.
13. Mallett AJ, McCarthy HJ, Ho G, Holman K, Farnsworth E, Patel C, Fletcher JT, Mallawaarachchi A, Quinlan C, Bennetts B, et al. Massively parallel sequencing and targeted exomes in familial kidney disease can diagnose underlying genetic disorders. Kidney Int. 2017;92(6):1493–506.
14. Connaughton DM, Kennedy C, Shril S, Mann N, Murray SL, Williams PA, Conlon E, Nakayama M, van der Ven AT, Ityel H. Monogenic causes of chronic kidney disease in adults. Kidney Int. 2019;95:914–28.
15. Nestor JG, Marasa M, Milo-Rasouly H, Groopman EE, Husain SA, Mohan S, Fernandez H, Aggarwal VS, Ahram DF, Vena N. Pilot study of return of genetic results to patients in adult nephrology. Clin J Am Soc Nephrol. 2020;15:651–64.
16. Snoek R, Van Setten J, Keating BJ, Israni AK, Jacobson PA, Oetting WS, Matas AJ, Mannon RB, Zhang Z, Zhang W. NPHP1 (Nephrocystin-1) gene deletions cause adult-onset ESRD. J Am Soc Nephrol. 2018;29:1772–9.
17. Cornec-Le Gall E, Audrézet M-P, Chen J-M, Hourmant M, Morin M-P, Perrichot R, Charasse C, Whebe B, Renaudineau E, Jousset P. Type of PKD1 mutation influences renal outcome in ADPKD. J Am Soc Nephrol. 2013;24:1006–13.
18. Torres VE, Chapman AB, Devuyst O, Gansevoort RT, Perrone RD, Koch G, Ouyang J, McQuade RD, Blais JD, Czerwiec FS. Tolvaptan in later-stage autosomal dominant polycystic kidney disease. N Engl J Med. 2017;377:1930–42.
19. Chebib FT, Perrone RD, Chapman AB, Dahl NK, Harris PC, Mrug M, Mustafa RA, Rastogi A, Watnick T, Alan S. A practical guide for treatment of rapidly progressive ADPKD with tolvaptan. J Am Soc Nephrol. 2018;29:2458–70.
20. De Wert G. Preimplantation genetic diagnosis: the ethics of intermediate cases. Hum Reprod. 2005;20:3261–6.
21. Malone AF, Phelan PJ, Hall G, Cetincelik U, Homstad A, Alonso AS, Jiang R, Lindsey TB, Wu G, Sparks MA, et al. Rare hereditary COL4A3/COL4A4 variants may be mistaken for familial focal segmental glomerulosclerosis. Kidney Int. 2014;86:1253–9.
22. Gast C, Pengelly RJ, Lyon M, Bunyan DJ, Seaby EG, Graham N, Venkat-Raman G, Ennis S. Collagen (COL4A) mutations are the most frequent mutations underlying adult focal segmental glomerulosclerosis. Nephrol Dial Transplant. 2016;31:961–70.
23. Jais JP, Knebelmann B, Giatras I, De Marchi M, Rizzoni G, Renieri A, Weber M, Gross O, Netzer KO, Flinter F, et al. X-linked Alport syndrome: natural history and genotype-phenotype correlations in girls and women belonging to 195 families: a "European Community Alport Syndrome Concerted Action" study. J Am Soc Nephrol. 2003;14:2603–10.
24. Gross O, Netzer KO, Lambrecht R, Seibold S, Weber M. Meta-analysis of genotype-phenotype correlation in X-linked Alport syndrome: impact on clinical counselling. Nephrol Dial Transplant. 2002;17:1218–27.
25. Bekheirnia MR, Reed B, Gregory MC, McFann K, Shamshirsaz AA, Masoumi A, Schrier RW. Genotype-phenotype correlation in X-linked Alport syndrome. J Am Soc Nephrol. 2010;21:876–83.

26. Persikov AV, Pillitteri RJ, Amin P, Schwarze U, Byers PH, Brodsky B. Stability related bias in residues replacing glycines within the collagen triple helix (Gly-Xaa-Yaa) in inherited connective tissue disorders. Hum Mutat. 2004;24:330–7.
27. Tan R, Colville D, Wang YY, Rigby L, Savige J. Alport retinopathy results from "severe" COL4A5 mutations and predicts early renal failure. Clin J Am Soc Nephrol. 2010;5:34–8.
28. Savige J, Gregory M, Gross O, Kashtan C, Ding J, Flinter F. Expert guidelines for the management of Alport syndrome and thin basement membrane nephropathy. J Am Soc Nephrol. 2013;24:364–75.
29. Savige J, Ariani F, Mari F, Bruttini M, Renieri A, Gross O, Deltas C, Flinter F, Ding J, Gale DP, et al. Expert consensus guidelines for the genetic diagnosis of Alport syndrome. Pediatr Nephrol. 2019;34:1175–89.
30. Savige J, Sheth S, Leys A, Nicholson A, Mack HG, Colville D. Ocular features in Alport syndrome: pathogenesis and clinical significance. Clin J Am Soc Nephrol. 2015;10:703–9.
31. Temme J, Peters F, Lange K, Pirson Y, Heidet L, Torra R, Grunfeld JP, Weber M, Licht C, Muller GA, et al. Incidence of renal failure and nephroprotection by RAAS inhibition in heterozygous carriers of X-chromosomal and autosomal recessive Alport mutations. Kidney Int. 2012;81:779–83.
32. Gillion V, Dahan K, Cosyns J-P, Hilbert P, Jadoul M, Goffin E, Godefroid N, De Meyer M, Mourad M, Pirson Y. Genotype and outcome after kidney transplantation in Alport syndrome. Kidney Int Rep. 2018;3:652–60.
33. Kashtan CE. Renal transplantation in patients with Alport syndrome: patient selection, outcomes, and donor evaluation. Int J Nephrol Renov Dis. 2018;11:267.
34. Lepori N, Zand L, Sethi S, Fernandez-Juarez G, Fervenza FC. Clinical and pathological phenotype of genetic causes of focal segmental glomerulosclerosis in adults. Clin Kidney J. 2018;11:179–90.
35. De Vriese AS, Sethi S, Nath KA, Glassock RJ, Fervenza FC. Differentiating primary, genetic, and secondary FSGS in adults: a clinicopathologic approach. J Am Soc Nephrol. 2018;29:759–74.
36. D'Agati VD, Kaskel FJ, Falk RJ. Focal segmental glomerulosclerosis. N Engl J Med. 2011;365:2398–411.
37. Cocchi E, Nestor JG, Gharavi AG. Clinical genetic screening in adult patients with kidney disease. Clin J Am Soc Nephrol. 2020;15:1497–510.
38. Hinkes B, Wiggins RC, Gbadegesin R, Vlangos CN, Seelow D, Nürnberg G, Garg P, Verma R, Chaib H, Hoskins BE, et al. Positional cloning uncovers mutations in PLCE1 responsible for a nephrotic syndrome variant that may be reversible. Nat Genet. 2006;38:1397–405.
39. Sampson MG, Gillies CE, Robertson CC, Crawford B, Vega-Warner V, Otto EA, Kretzler M, Kang HM. Using population genetics to interrogate the monogenic nephrotic syndrome diagnosis in a case cohort. J Am Soc Nephrol. 2016;27:1970–83.
40. Morello W, Puvinathan S, Puccio G, Ghiggeri GM, Dello Strologo L, Peruzzi L, Murer L, Cioni M, Guzzo I, Cocchi E, et al. Post-transplant recurrence of steroid resistant nephrotic syndrome in children: the Italian experience. J Nephrol. 2019;33(4):849–57.
41. Ashraf S, Gee HY, Woerner S, Xie LX, Vega-Warner V, Lovric S, Fang H, Song X, Cattran DC, Avila-Casado C, et al. ADCK4 mutations promote steroid-resistant nephrotic syndrome through CoQ10 biosynthesis disruption. J Clin Invest. 2013;123:5179–89.
42. Diomedi-Camassei F, Di Giandomenico S, Santorelli FM, Caridi G, Piemonte F, Montini G, Ghiggeri GM, Murer L, Barisoni L, Pastore A, et al. COQ2 nephropathy: a newly described inherited mitochondriopathy with primary renal involvement. J Am Soc Nephrol. 2007;18:2773–80.
43. Montini G, Malaventura C, Salviati L. Early coenzyme Q10 supplementation in primary coenzyme Q10 deficiency. N Engl J Med. 2008;358:2849–50.
44. Rötig A, Appelkvist EL, Geromel V, Chretien D, Kadhom N, Edery P, Lebideau M, Dallner G, Munnich A, Ernster L, et al. Quinone-responsive multiple respiratory-chain dysfunction due to widespread coenzyme Q10 deficiency. Lancet. 2000;356:391–5.

45. Rheault MN, Savige J, Randles MJ, Weinstock A, Stepney M, Turner AN, Parziale G, Gross O, Flinter FA, Miner JH, et al. The importance of clinician, patient and researcher collaborations in Alport syndrome. Pediatr Nephrol. 2020;35:733–42.
46. Wang M, Chun J, Genovese G, Knob AU, Benjamin A, Wilkins MS, Friedman DJ, Appel GB, Lifton RP, Mane S, et al. Contributions of rare gene variants to familial and sporadic FSGS. J Am Soc Nephrol. 2019;30:1625–40.
47. Lovric S, Ashraf S, Tan W, Hildebrandt F. Genetic testing in steroid-resistant nephrotic syndrome: when and how? Nephrol Dial Transplant. 2016;31:1802–13.
48. Breslow NE, Collins AJ, Ritchey ML, Grigoriev YA, Peterson SM, Green DM. End stage renal disease in patients with Wilms tumor: results from the National Wilms Tumor Study Group and the United States Renal Data System. J Urol. 2005;174:1972–5.
49. Nadkarni GN, Galarneau G, Ellis SB, Nadukuru R, Zhang J, Scott SA, Schurmann C, Li R, Rasmussen-Torvik LJ, Kho AN. Apolipoprotein L1 variants and blood pressure traits in African Americans. J Am Coll Cardiol. 2017;69:1564–74.
50. Zahr R, Lebensburger J, Rampersaud E, Hankins JS, Estepp JH. Children with sickle cell anemia and APOL1 gene variants develop albuminuria early in life. Blood. 2018;132:2377.
51. Freedman BI, Langefeld CD, Andringa KK, Croker JA, Williams AH, Garner NE, Birmingham DJ, Hebert LA, Hicks PJ, Segal MS. End-stage renal disease in African Americans with lupus nephritis is associated with APOL1. Arthritis Rheumatol. 2014;66:390–6.
52. Fine DM, Wasser WG, Estrella MM, Atta MG, Kuperman M, Shemer R, Rajasekaran A, Tzur S, Racusen LC, Skorecki K. APOL1 risk variants predict histopathology and progression to ESRD in HIV-related kidney disease. J Am Soc Nephrol. 2012;23:343–50.
53. Wu H, Larsen CP, Hernandez-Arroyo CF, Mohamed MM, Caza T, Sharshir MD, Chughtai A, Xie L, Gimenez JM, Sandow TA. AKI and collapsing glomerulopathy associated with COVID-19 and APOL1 high-risk genotype. J Am Soc Nephrol. 2020;31:1688–95.
54. Genovese G, Friedman DJ, Ross MD, Lecordier L, Uzureau P, Freedman BI, Bowden DW, Langefeld CD, Oleksyk TK, Knob ALU. Association of trypanolytic ApoL1 variants with kidney disease in African Americans. Science. 2010;329:841–5.
55. Freedman BI, Locke JE, Reeves-Daniel AM, Julian BA. Apolipoprotein L1 gene effects on kidney transplantation. In: Seminars in nephrology. Amsterdam: Elsevier; 2017. p. 530–7.
56. Mohan S, Iltis AS, Sawinski D, DuBois JM. APOL1 genetic testing in living kidney transplant donors. Am J Kidney Dis. 2019;74:538–43.
57. Wang XV, Blades N, Ding J, Sultana R, Parmigiani G. Estimation of sequencing error rates in short reads. BMC Bioinf. 2012;13:185.
58. Sen ES, Dean P, Yarram-Smith L, Bierzynska A, Woodward G, Buxton C, Dennis G, Welsh GI, Williams M, Saleem MA. Clinical genetic testing using a custom-designed steroid-resistant nephrotic syndrome gene panel: analysis and recommendations. J Med Genet. 2017;54:795–804.
59. Bullich G, Domingo-Gallego A, Vargas I, Ruiz P, Lorente-Grandoso L, Furlano M, Fraga G, Madrid Á, Ariceta G, Borregán M. A kidney-disease gene panel allows a comprehensive genetic diagnosis of cystic and glomerular inherited kidney diseases. Kidney Int. 2018;94:363–71.
60. Groopman EE, Marasa M, Cameron-Christie S, Petrovski S, Aggarwal VS, Milo-Rasouly H, Li Y, Zhang J, Nestor J, Krithivasan P, et al. Diagnostic utility of exome sequencing for kidney disease. N Engl J Med. 2019;380:142–51.
61. Xue Y, Ankala A, Wilcox WR, Hegde MR. Solving the molecular diagnostic testing conundrum for Mendelian disorders in the era of next-generation sequencing: single-gene, gene panel, or exome/genome sequencing. Genet Med. 2015;17:444–51.
62. Vivante A, Hwang DY, Kohl S, Chen J, Shril S, Schulz J, van der Ven A, Daouk G, Soliman NA, Kumar AS, et al. Exome sequencing discerns syndromes in patients from consanguineous families with congenital anomalies of the kidneys and urinary tract. J Am Soc Nephrol. 2017;28:69–75.

63. Warejko JK, Tan W, Daga A, Schapiro D, Lawson JA, Shril S, Lovric S, Ashraf S, Rao J, Hermle T, et al. Whole exome sequencing of patients with steroid-resistant nephrotic syndrome. Clin J Am Soc Nephrol. 2018;13:53–62.
64. van der Ven AT, Connaughton DM, Ityel H, Mann N, Nakayama M, Chen J, Vivante A, Hwang DY, Schulz J, Braun DA, et al. Whole-exome sequencing identifies causative mutations in families with congenital anomalies of the kidney and urinary tract. J Am Soc Nephrol. 2018;29:2348–61.
65. Mann N, Braun DA, Amann K, Tan W, Shril S, Connaughton DM, Nakayama M, Schneider R, Kitzler TM, van der Ven AT, et al. Whole-exome sequencing enables a precision medicine approach for kidney transplant recipients. J Am Soc Nephrol. 2019;30:201–15.
66. Lata S, Marasa M, Li Y, Fasel DA, Groopman E, Jobanputra V, Rasouly H, Mitrotti A, Westland R, Verbitsky M, et al. Whole-exome sequencing in adults with chronic kidney disease: a pilot study. Ann Intern Med. 2018;168:100–9.
67. Rao J, Liu X, Mao J, Tang X, Shen Q, Li G, Sun L, Bi Y, Wang X, Qian Y, et al. Genetic spectrum of renal disease for 1001 Chinese children based on a multicenter registration system. Clin Genet. 2019;96:402–10.
68. Sadowski CE, Lovric S, Ashraf S, Pabst WL, Gee HY, Kohl S, Engelmann S, Vega-Warner V, Fang H, Halbritter J, et al. A single-gene cause in 29.5% of cases of steroid-resistant nephrotic syndrome. J Am Soc Nephrol. 2015;26:1279–89.
69. Bierzynska A, McCarthy HJ, Soderquest K, Sen ES, Colby E, Ding WY, Nabhan MM, Kerecuk L, Hegde S, Hughes D, et al. Genomic and clinical profiling of a national nephrotic syndrome cohort advocates a precision medicine approach to disease management. Kidney Int. 2017;91(4):937–47.
70. Gribouval O, Boyer O, Hummel A, Dantal J, Martinez F, Sberro-Soussan R, Etienne I, Chauveau D, Delahousse M, Lionet A, et al. Identification of genetic causes for sporadic steroid-resistant nephrotic syndrome in adults. Kidney Int. 2018;94:1013–22.
71. Marchesin V, Pérez-Martí A, Le Meur G, Pichler R, Grand K, Klootwijk ED, Kesselheim A, Kleta R, Lienkamp S, Simons M. Molecular basis for autosomal-dominant renal Fanconi syndrome caused by HNF4A. Cell Rep. 2019;29:4407–21.
72. Birdwell KA, Decker B, Barbarino JM, Peterson JF, Stein CM, Sadee W, Wang D, Vinks AA, He Y, Swen JJ, et al. Clinical pharmacogenetics implementation consortium (CPIC) guidelines for CYP3A5 genotype and tacrolimus dosing. Clin Pharmacol Therap. 2015;98:19–24.

Chapter 2
Application of Artificial Intelligence and Machine Learning in Kidney Disease

Caitlin Monaghan, Kristina Looper, and Len Usvyat

Artificial Intelligence and Machine Learning

Artificial intelligence (AI) is a broad field of computer science focused on studying and creating intelligent machines. In this context, there are several possible definitions for determining what "intelligence" means: one can consider whether a machine thinks or behaves like a human, or whether it thinks or behaves rationally, when determining whether it is intelligent [1]. In a practical sense, this means creating a computer system that can sense things about the world around it and make decisions based on that information. The decision made will be determined by the goals the AI system was designed for.

From this definition, we can consider an AI system as a "rational agent" that can use sensors to gather data about its environment and then act in or on that environment with actuators [1]. The input data from the sensor will be processed by some form of decision-making algorithm to determine its behavior. A diagram of such a system can be seen in Fig. 2.1.

AI has a variety of subfields dedicated to understanding different types of input. Some examples are computer vision for teaching a computer to "see" images, natural language processing for understanding human language, and speech recognition for understanding spoken language [2].

Machine learning (ML) is a subfield of AI, focusing on the decision-making algorithm portion of the system. It focuses on using data-driven methods to allow the AI to learn about the environment from which it is getting data and improve the model driving its decisions [3]. The process of providing data to an ML algorithm to allow it to learn is called "training." The goal of training is to produce a high-performing

C. Monaghan · K. Looper · L. Usvyat (✉)
Fresenius Medical Care, Waltham, MA, USA
e-mail: Caitlin.Monaghan@freseniusmedicalcare.com;
Len.Usvyat@freseniusmedicalcare.com

S. J. Saggi, M. O. Salifu (eds.), *Technological Advances in Care of Patients with Kidney Diseases*, https://doi.org/10.1007/978-3-031-11942-2_2

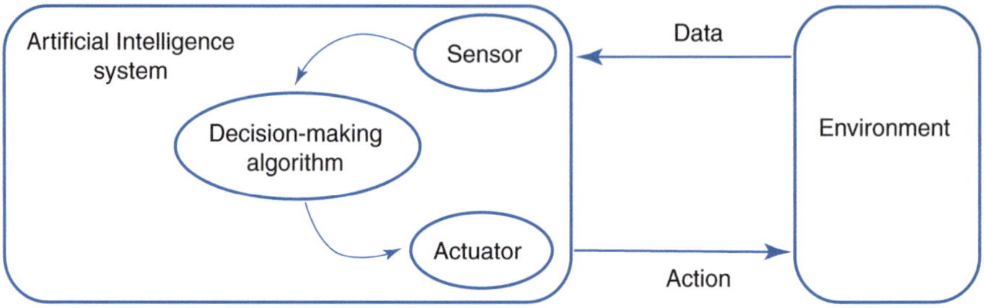

Fig. 2.1 A diagram of the components of an artificial intelligence system

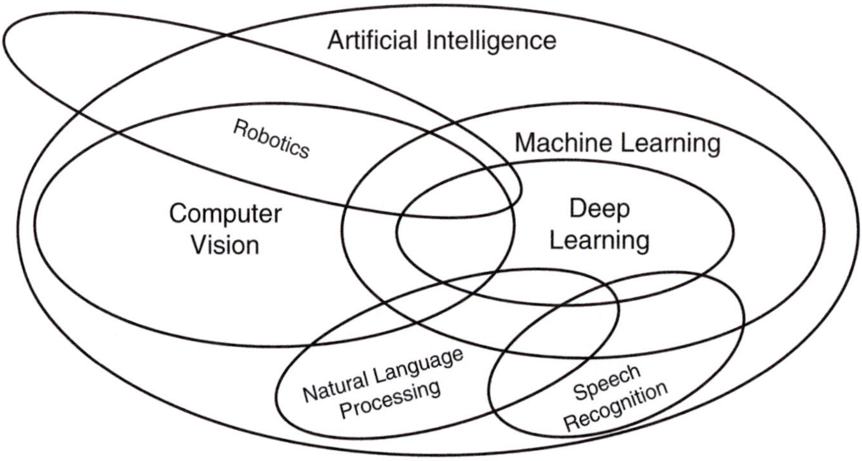

Fig. 2.2 Relationship between artificial intelligence, machine learning, deep learning, and other related fields. Figure provided by Prof. Justin Johnson

model that can perform its given task in a way that generalizes well to new input data [4]. In traditional ML applications, features are selected or extracted from the input data to help aid the training process. The set of methods called "representation learning" provide ways to give raw data to a machine and allow it to select its own features. Deep learning is a type of representation learning with several processing layers creating several levels of representations [5]. Figure 2.2 shows the relationship between AI, ML, deep learning, and other related fields.

The method of providing or the presence of ground truth when building an ML algorithm defines the class of learning it falls under. There are three main types: supervised learning, unsupervised learning, and reinforcement learning [1]. Predictive modeling problems are typically solved with supervised learning, though unsupervised learning methods are often used to reduce the dimension of the data's input features. In supervised learning, the input data is labeled with a target variable to be predicted. This target variable can be a discrete category, like learning whether an image is a cat or a dog, or a continuous variable, like predicting someone's height. If the target variable of a supervised learning model consists of discrete classes, this is called "classification" problem; if it is a continuous variable, it is a "regression" problem. Some common examples of supervised learning algorithms are linear regression, logistic regression, support vector machines, and neural networks [6].

In unsupervised learning, the data do not contain a labeled target variable. Instead, the learning algorithm finds a way of concisely describing the data. Examples of this are clustering, which attempts to find groupings with similar features inside of the data, or anomaly detection, which can detect data that are unusual [1, 3]. Reinforcement learning algorithms are goal-oriented algorithms that learn by trial and error from their environment. When the algorithm performs an action, it is rewarded for performing it correctly and learns from that feedback [7].

In recent years, work in the field of deep neural networks has led to major progress in modeling problems in a variety of domains, including image analysis and genomics [5]. Versions of neural network models, such as convolutional neural networks and recurrent neural networks, have provided state-of-the-art performance in the fields of computer vision and speech recognition.

Data and ESKD

The more data that exist for a patient, the greater is our ability to assess a patient's condition. Kidney disease is a unique area of health care where patient-related data are abundant. This is especially true as patients transition to ESKD with frequent in-center or home dialysis treatments and frequent lab collections; their dialysis provider's electronic health record (EHR) becomes an amalgamation of all patient-related information.

Large and small dialysis organizations have collected significant amounts of patient treatment data. These data are extraordinarily detailed with hundreds of data elements collected per treatment, many on a per second interval. Some of these data elements are very structured, such as pure numbers in a tabular format, while others are not structured. In fact, data come in a variety of ways beyond numeric, including images, text, paper, videos, and multimedia.

Traditional clinical data described above, typically collected through EHRs or claims, contain demographic information, clinical parameters, medical history, procedures, and medications, but this may be insufficient to deliver a complete numeric fingerprint of the patient. Just as it is impossible to accurately understand the geography of a certain region without looking at various layers of information about it, it is similarly impossible to build a complete story about a patient without seeing clinical data supplemented with information from other sources [8]. Aggregating clinical data with additional data sources makes it actionable and insightful [9, 10].

What are some of these data sources? Some have existed for many years while others are becoming available through new technology and shared public information (Fig. 2.3). Weather forecast data collected through various cloud computing vendors can help us understand the climate and environment where patients live and

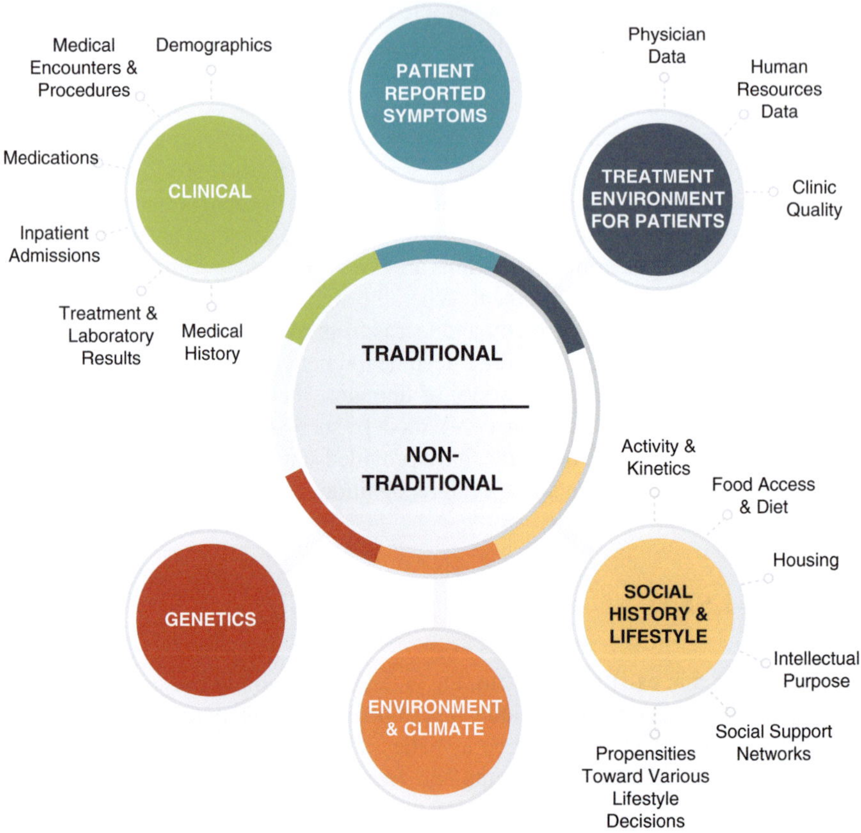

Fig. 2.3 Traditional and non-traditional examples of data sources

can be used in predicting when patients are more likely to miss dialysis treatments [11]. Census data, which have been electronically available since the late 1990s, assist in identifying which patients live in areas with low household incomes or large household sizes, for example.

Novel, non-clinical data sources are actively being created. For example, to understand a patient's kinetic activity, walkability scores may help [12]. Data on proximity to grocery stores, hospitals, urgent care facilities, and civic center institutions available through Google Maps can aid in understanding a patient's home environment. During the COVID-19 pandemic, highly localized data on COVID-19 outbreaks may be helpful in predicting what would happen to dialysis populations.

In addition to utilizing geography-level data sources, real-time data are essential. We can understand patient movement and sleep patterns by using real-time data from fitness trackers and sensors and this has already proven useful in understanding patient outcomes [12–14].

Data from multiple sources provide a truly well-rounded view of the patient, yet data alone are not sufficient to create a coherent, actionable patient story; we need ways of putting the story together through data analytics to deliver actionable insights.

AI Applications in Kidney Disease

Despite the unique abundance of data generated during the standard care of hemodialysis patients, the number of applications of AI and ML in kidney disease have lagged in comparison to other specialties such as oncology or cardiology. However, now that other disciplines have clearly benefitted from AI support, the presence of AI in nephrology is growing in ways both common across fields and in use cases unique to ESKD.

AI-enabled applications supporting diagnostics or predicting a patient's current state as it relates to diagnoses, commonly span multiple data types, including images, tabular data, and unstructured data. The field of radiology has seen an explosion of AI tools developed to aid in assessing medical images, particularly using computer vision techniques to identify the presence of abnormalities both quickly and accurately. While medical images are typically outside the scope of routinely collected data, smart phones can be used to easily and noninvasively capture and grade vascular access aneurysms with over 90% classification accuracy [15]. Within the scope of utilizing routinely collected data to aid in diagnostics, ML predictive models can be utilized to identify dialysis patients with a variety of ailments, such as active COVID-19 infections, by using typical laboratory and treatment measures [16].

ML also excels in predicting the risk of events yet to happen. Appropriately, a large amount of work has focused on first year mortality in various ESKD populations, such as individuals starting HD [17, 18], patients with pediatric dialysis starts [19], and those on peritoneal dialysis (PD) [20], which can help guide treatment choices and care. Additionally, ML has been employed to predict PD technique failure [21] and the appearance of hypotension during hemodialysis treatment [22, 23].

Complex relationships, such as those involved in medication management, can also be modeled through ML algorithms. Anemia management in ESKD can be a challenging problem in many hemodialysis patients where hemoglobin values must be maintained within narrow targets through erythropoiesis-stimulating agent (ESA) and iron dosing. Barbieri and colleagues have reported on the development and implementation of a predictive model to aid in ESA and iron administration [24, 25]. They built an artificial neural network to predict hemoglobin concentrations 3 months ahead using information from the medical record and subsequent 90-day ESA/iron prescription with a mean absolute error of 0.75 g/dL, with much of the error attributable to unpredictable events [24]. When implemented in clinics, use of their anemia control model (ACM) resulted in decreased ESA consumption, increased on-target hemoglobin values, and decreased in individual patient hemoglobin fluctuations [25].

Conclusion

AI and ML solutions together with technology-driven advancements led to significant improvements in care delivery paradigms. Nephrology and kidney disease, while lagging other fields such as oncology and cardiology, is also advancing in providing data-driven solutions. Most of the advancements in kidney disease occurred in patients with ESKD. This is because of the richness of the data that are obtained through routine home and in-center dialysis treatments.

Ethical considerations are important factors in making sure that no biases are introduced with AI solutions. Some examples of biases have occurred when historical data used to build predictive models are biased; for instance, historically, patients living in smaller housing units may have been less likely to dialyze at home, but with newer and more compact home dialysis technologies this is less of a concern.

AI solutions should not be built independently from clinical care pathways. More integrated solutions incorporating AI at the dialysis chair is important. We believe that AI solutions should be done in compliment with clinical judgement of doctors, nurses, dietitians, social workers, and technicians working with patients. Most robust AI solutions are those that properly rely on both the clinical staff decision making as well as computer-driven AI algorithms.

We expect advancement in technologies—including cloud computing, increases in the amount of data collected through multiple sensors, and newer modeling methods in statistics, mathematics, and computer science—will lead to continued incremental improvements in how care to patients with kidney disease is delivered.

References

1. Norvig P. Artificial intelligence: a modern approach. Hoboken: Prentice Hall; 2009.
2. Johnson J. Presented as part of EECS 498-007: deep learning for computer vision. Available from: https://youtu.be/dJYGatp4SvA.
3. Barber D. Bayesian reasoning and machine learning. Cambridge: Cambridge University Press; 2012.
4. Bishop C. Pattern recognition and machine learning. Cham: Springer; 2006.
5. LeCun Y, Bengio Y, Hinton G. Deep learning. Nature. 2015;521(7553):436–44.
6. Kuhn M. Applied predictive modeling. Cham: Springer; 2013.
7. Sutton RSBA. Reinforcement learning: an introduction. 2nd ed. Cambridge: MIT Press; 2018.
8. Hawgood S, Hook-Barnard IG, O'Brien TC, Yamamoto KR. Precision medicine: beyond the inflection point. Sci Transl Med. 2015;7:300.

9. Data-driven healthcare organizations use big data analytics for big gains. Available at: https://www-03.ibm.com/industries/ca/en/healthcare/documents/Data_driven_healthcare_organizations_use_big_data_analytics_for_big_gains.pdf. Accessed January 30, 2018.
10. 5 Reasons healthcare data is unique and difficult to measure. Available at: https://www.healthcatalyst.com/5-reasons-healthcare-data-is-difficult-to-measure. Accessed January 30, 2018.
11. Jiao Y, Brzozowski J, Zhang H, Kuang Z, Conti J, Chaudhuri S. Testing of prediction models for end stage kidney disease patient nonadherence to renal replacement treatment regimens. In: Women in statistics and data science conference, Charlotte, NC, 2016.
12. Larkin JW, Han M, Williams S, Ye X, Usvyat LA, Kotanko P, et al. Relationship of neighborhood walkability and dialysis patient characteristics and outcomes. New Orleans: American Society of Nephrology Kidney; 2017.
13. Antman EM, Benjamin EJ, Harrington RA, Houser SR, Peterson ED, Bauman MA, et al. Acquisition, analysis, and sharing of data in 2015 and beyond: a survey of the landscape: a conference report from the American Heart Association Data Summit 2015. J Am Heart Assoc. 2015;4:11.
14. Han M, Preciado P, Thwin O, Tao X, Tapia-Silva LM, Fuentes LR, et al. Effect of statewide lockdown in response to COVID-19 pandemic on physical activity levels of hemodialysis patients. Blood Purif. 2021;2021:1–8.
15. Krackov W, Sor M, Razdan R, Zheng H, Kotanko P. Artificial intelligence methods for rapid vascular access aneurysm classification in remote or in-person settings. Blood Purif. 2021;2021:1–6.
16. Monaghan CK, Larkin JW, Chaudhuri S, Han H, Jiao Y, Bermudez KM, et al. Machine learning for prediction of patients on hemodialysis with an undetected SARS-CoV-2 infection. Kidney. 2021;2:456–68.
17. Akbilgic O, Obi Y, Potukuchi PK, Karabayir I, Nguyen DV, Soohoo M, et al. Machine learning to identify dialysis patients at high death risk. Kidney Int Rep. 2019;4:1219–29.
18. Sheng K, Zhang P, Yao X, Li J, He Y, Chen J. Prognostic machine learning models for first-year mortality in incident hemodialysis patients: development and validation study. JMIR Med Inform. 2020;8:1–11.
19. Gotta V, Tancev G, Marsenic O, Vogt JE, Pfister M. Identifying key predictors of mortality in young patients on chronic haemodialysis-a machine learning approach. Nephrol Dial Transplant. 2021;36:519–28.
20. Noh J, Yoo KD, Bae W, Lee JS, Kim K, Cho JH, et al. Prediction of the mortality risk in peritoneal dialysis patients using machine learning models: a nation-wide prospective cohort in Korea. Sci Rep. 2020;10:1–11.
21. Tangri N, Ansell D, Naimark D. Predicting technique survival in peritoneal dialysis patients: comparing artificial neural networks and logistic regression. Nephrol Dial Transplant. 2008;23:2972–81.
22. Barbieri C, Cattinelli I, Neri L, Mari F, Ramos R, Brancaccio D, et al. Development of an artificial intelligence model to guide the management of blood pressure, fluid volume, and dialysis dose in end-stage kidney disease patients: proof of concept and first clinical assessment. Kidney Dis. 2019;5:28–33.
23. Gómez-Pulido JA, Gómez-Pulido JM, Rodríguez-Puyol D, Polo-Luque ML, Vargas-Lombardo M. Predicting the appearance of hypotension during hemodialysis sessions using machine learning classifiers. Int J Environ Res Public Health. 2021;18:1–17.
24. Barbieri C, Bolzoni E, Mari F, Cattinelli I, Bellocchio F, Martin JD, et al. Performance of a predictive model for long-term hemoglobin response to darbepoetin and iron administration in a large cohort of hemodialysis patients. PLoS ONE. 2016;11:1–18.
25. Barbieri C, Molina M, Ponce P, Tothova M, Cattinelli I, Ion Titapiccolo J, et al. An international observational study suggests that artificial intelligence for clinical decision support optimizes anemia management in hemodialysis patients. Kidney Int. 2016;90:422–9.

Chapter 3
The Role of The Metabolism/Exposome in Chronic Kidney Disease: Discovery for Precision Nutrition

Wimal Pathmasiri, Madison Schroder, Susan McRitchie, and Susan Sumner

Need of Novel Biomarkers for Chronic Kidney Disease

Chronic kidney disease (CKD) impacts between 8% and 16% of the population in the world [1]. CKD has become one of the prominent causes of death globally [2]. Type 1 diabetes (T1D), Type 2 diabetes (T2D), and blood pressure (high or low) are the major comorbidities associated with CKD [3], and it is known that nearly 1/3 of diabetic patients develop CKD [3]. The CKD diagnosis depends on the chronic reduction in kidney function and structural kidney damage [4].

According to the current international guidelines, CKD is defined as a decrease in kidney function shown by reduced glomerular filtration rate (GFR) or one or more of the following markers: albuminuria; urinary sediment abnormality; electrolyte or other abnormality due to tubular disorder; abnormalities on histology; structural abnormalities detected by imaging; history of kidney transplantation) of kidney damage or both for at least 3 months regardless of the underlying cause [4]. CKD is classified into categories or stages (G1, G2, G3a, G3b, G4, and G5), where G5 is the end-stage renal disease (ESRD) [4]. GFR is estimated (eGFR) based on the serum creatinine level of an individual using clinical equations (Modification of Diet in Renal Disease (MDRD), study equation, and Chronic Kidney Disease Epidemiology (CKD-EPI) equation) [5]. It has become evident that these equations are not reliable because they fail to provide an accurate estimate of GFR in situations frequently encountered in clinical practice. The use of eGFR for the diagnosis of CKD is insufficient to determine the cause of kidney injury, due to the complexity of CKD and its comorbidities.

W. Pathmasiri (✉) · M. Schroder · S. McRitchie · S. Sumner
Department of Nutrition, Nutrition Research Institute, University of North Carolina at Chapel Hill, Chapel Hill, NC, USA
e-mail: wimal_pathmasiri@unc.edu; schrodm@email.unc.edu; susan_mcritchie@unc.edu; susan_sumner@unc.edu

S. J. Saggi, M. O. Salifu (eds.), *Technological Advances in Care of Patients with Kidney Diseases*, https://doi.org/10.1007/978-3-031-11942-2_3

Many individuals are asymptomatic of their CKD until they have progressed to advanced stages of the disease [4, 6]. Extensive pathological examinations using tissue biopsies or imaging techniques are needed to confirm the disease stage and the extent of the kidney damage. Renal biopsy is an invasive method, while tissue imaging methods are expensive. These methods are impractical for the early diagnosis of CKD, particularly in cohorts who do not have access to advanced medical care.

There is an urgent need for developing novel biomarkers in relatively non-invasive biofluids that can more precisely identify individuals at risk for CKD development, before or in the early stages of developing CKD, while also providing information on the stage and disease etiology of CKD.

Consequently, developing novel biomarkers for early detection and treatment of CKD is crucial for clinicians to mitigate adverse clinical outcomes, including ESRD, cardiovascular disease, and increased mortality. Recent advances in high throughput omics technologies (genomics, transcriptomics, proteomics, metabolomics, metallomics [7], and exposomics) [8, 9] in combination with data analytics methods (e.g., statistics, chemometrics, bioinformatics, and machine learning) [10–12] will significantly facilitate discovering new biomarkers, especially when applying approaches that integrate these multi-omics data. The following sections explore some technologies and biomarker studies in CKD.

Metabotype and Metabolomics Analysis

Metabolomics involves the systematic measure of the low molecular weight complement of cells, tissues, feces, and biological fluids. The metabotype (metabolic phenotype) of an individual is the metabolic signature or the biochemical fingerprint of low molecular weight metabolites that are present at any time in given tissues or biological fluids [13]. The metabolic fingerprint comprises a total collection of metabolites (metabolome) that includes endogenous metabolites derived from the host system (i.e., those that map to biochemical pathways of the host) and exogenous metabolites derived from exposures (e.g., dietary intake, supplements, medications, environmental chemicals) [14, 15]. The ability to assess individuals' metabotypes and to understand variation in metabotypes across clinical and epidemiological cohorts allows the discovery of metabolic biomarkers of disease risk across demographics and populations, and to reveal metabotypes associated with patient management and outcomes [15, 16].

Commonly used biospecimens in metabolomics investigations include relatively non-invasive biological fluids (e.g., urine, plasma, serum, umbilical cord blood, and plasma), excreta (e.g., urine, feces, sweat, and breath), invasive fluids (cerebral spinal fluid), and organ tissue (e.g., muscle, liver, kidney, and brain) that are rich in low molecular weight metabolites. Analysis of samples from model systems and human subject investigations have shown that the metabotype is correlated with factors such as genetic composition [17] (e.g., gender, age, ethnicity, genetic polymorphisms), environmental exposures (e.g., medications, illicit drugs, environmental pollutants, contaminants in food and water), lifestyle factors (e.g., tobacco use, exercise, stress, diet), gut microbes, physical and clinical phenotypes (e.g., height, weight, blood pressure, heart rate), mental health status (e.g., depression, cognitive scores), dietary intake and nutrient status, and many disease states [18, 19]. Therefore, it is necessary to consider these factors when designing metabolomic studies.

The terms metabolomics, metabonomics, metabolic profiling, metabolic phenotyping, and metabotyping are widely used interchangeably by the research community [15, 16, 20–23]. Metabotyping biospecimens obtained from humans or model systems provide a means to reveal patterns, specific metabolites involved, pathway perturbations associated with health and disease, associated genetic determinants, and to inform treatment/intervention strategies. Studies that involve metabolomics can be designed to uncover biomarkers that are associated with specific study phenotypes, such as health or disease states, diet, exercise, or responsivity to treatment or intervention options. These research study designs address the need to develop more sensitive and early markers for disease diagnosis and staging, for monitoring treatment efficacy, for identifying adverse response or relapse or for examining the outcome of intervention strategies. Once marker metabolites associated with the study phenotypes are discovered, pathway mapping can be used to gain mechanistic insights to identifying potential targets for pharmacological development, for nutritional intervention, or to point to genetic polymorphisms. Studies must be designed to ensure that the link between the metabolomics profiles and the phenotypic anchors are not biased by factors that are known to correlate with the metabotype [17], and that the study is sufficiently powered considering the heterogeneity of the study population.

Targeted and Untargeted Metabolomics Analysis

Targeted metabolomics and untargeted metabolomics are terms used to define a selection of analytical data capture methodologies [9, 13] to analyze the metabolome. The targeted metabolomics analysis [24] involves the measurement of chemically characterized and biochemically annotated metabolites to address specific hypotheses, normally focused on metabolites in a particular pathway. For example, targeted metabolomics analysis of trimethylamine-N-oxide and related metabolites using liquid chromatography mass spectrometry (LC-MS) was used to determine the contribution of trimethylamine-N-oxide (TMAO) to inflammation and mortality in chronic kidney disease [25] (described in section, Influence of microbiome in CKD). Another example of targeted metabolomics analysis was an investigation aimed at the analysis of a set of metabolites by LC/MS to test the hypothesis that CKD progression and severity would impact the plasma concentrations and urinary excretion of amino acids [26].

Untargeted metabolomics is a method that is not necessarily focused on any specific hypotheses, but rather used to capture signals derived from a wide range of analytes, covering a variety of chemical classes and biological pathways [13, 18, 19]. In untargeted analysis, the endogenous counterpart of the metabolomics signatures (endometabolome) is composed of thousands of signals that belong to chemical classes such as amino acids, aromatic amino acids, biogenic amines, sugars, polysaccharides, phospholipids, sphingolipids, carnitines, catecholamines, purines, pyrimidines, hormones, and steroids, etc. In addition, untargeted platforms also enable the simultaneous capture of signals for metabolites of medications, illicit drugs, cosmetics and personal products, environmentally relevant chemicals, additives in foods, and compounds derived from the ingestion of foods (exometabolome). Nuclear magnetic resonance (NMR) spectroscopy and mass spectrometry (gas chromatography and liquid chromatography mass spectrometry (GC-MS and LC-MS) are used in untargeted metabolomics investigations [18, 19]. The higher resolution and sensitivity of mass spectroscopy (compared with NMR) enables the capture of signals for thousands of metabolites simultaneously [9]. NMR and GC- and LC-chromatography coupled mass spectrometry methods, as well as electrochemical detection (for detecting neuro transmitters) [27] or capillary electrophoresis methods [28] are employed in metabolomics investigations.

Standard statistical analysis methods (e.g., t-test; Mann–Whitney U test, and Wilcoxon test) are used to determine significance or fold change for signals, (peaks or features) between and amongst study phenotypes to reveal potential biomarkers [9, 13]. Supervised and unsupervised multivariate statistics methods are used to identify patterns of metabolite signals (or sets of markers) and their rank order of importance in defining study phenotypes. These signals are then identified through library matching to in-house physical standards libraries or annotated using public databases. These identified and annotated metabolites can be mapped to biochemical pathways, and other omics data can also be integrated through pathway mapping or network analysis to point to potential perturbations in metabolism that are associated with the study phenotypes. Targeted analysis approaches are needed to confirm or validate the discovery findings, by using biospecimens from external cohorts, or conducting well defined studies in appropriate in vivo or in vitro models [29]. In addition, stable isotopes can be used to confirm specific metabolic pathways, metabolic flux, and underlying mechanisms [30]. High throughput, high resolution analytical technologies and data analysis platforms have allowed for metabotyping in large scale population-based Metabolome Wide Association Studies (MWAS), metabolite-GWAS (mGWAS), and metabotype quantitative trait locus (mQTL) mapping studies by using both NMR Spectroscopy [31–33] and mass spectrometry [34–36]. Additional bioinformatics and data analytic approaches enhance identifying marker metabolic features or metabolites in biological samples from participants in properly designed cohort studies or from studies that involve animal or cell models. Each of these methods and approaches can be applied to discovering novel biomarker for disease risk of CKD.

Genetic Variations in CKD and Relationship to Proteins and Metabolites

Risk of disease is dependent on a number of factors or causes (socio-economic, demographic, cultural, environmental and genetic factors). Moreover, understanding of the genetic determinants of disease risk has greatly advanced with the introduction of genome-wide association studies (GWAS) [37] in large populations. Sandholm et al. [38] performed a GWAS study in a cohort of 3652 patients from the Finnish Diabetic Nephropathy Study (FinnDiane) with T1D and determined sex-specific genetic risk factors for ESRD exist. A common variant, rs4972593 on chromosome 2q31.1, was found to be associated with ESRD in females in this investigation. This association had been replicated in the meta-analysis of three independent T1D cohorts and remained to be significant for women after combined meta-analysis of the discovery and replication cohorts. The variant rs4972593 is located between the genes coding for the Sp3 transcription factor, which interacts directly with estrogen receptor α and is known to regulate the expression of genes linked to glomerular function and the pathogenesis of nephropathy, and the CDCA7 transcription factor, which regulates cell proliferation. Further analysis revealed potential transcription factor–binding sites within rs4972593 and predicted eight estrogen-responsive elements within 5 kb of this locus. In addition, sex-specific differences were found in the glomerular expression levels of SP3. These results indicate that the variant rs4972593 is a sex-specific genetic variant associated with ESRD in patients with T1D which may underlie the sex-specific protection against ESRD.

Kottgen et al. [39] conducted a GWAS to identify susceptibility loci for GFR, estimated by serum creatinine (eGFRcrea) and cystatin C (eGFRcys), and CKD (eGFRcrea <60 ml/min/1.73 m^2) in European-ancestry participants of four population-based cohorts (ARIC, CHS, FHS, RS; n = 19,877; 2388 CKD cases), and tested for replication in 21,466 participants (1932 CKD cases). Authors reported that significant single nucleotide polymorphisms (SNP) associations with CKD were identified at the UMOD locus, with eGFRcrea at UMOD, SHROOM3 and GATM-SPATA5L1, and with eGFRcys at CST and STC1. UMOD is known to encode the most common protein in human urine, Tamm-Horsfall protein2, and rare mutations in UMOD cause mendelian forms of kidney disease. These findings provide insights into CKD pathogenesis and underscore the importance of common genetic variants influencing renal function and disease.

Exposome and CKD

Studying genome and/or its downstream products (proteins, endogenous metabolites) alone is insufficient for understanding chronic diseases such as CKD. Risk factors for CKD development and progression could include an array of lifestyle and environmental triggers [8], such as body weight, exercise, dietary intake, tobacco use, and environmental chemicals. Many of these non-genetic factors can be discovered by analyzing the exposome.

The exposome is defined as the total measure of an individual's lifelong environmental exposure which complements to the genome [40–42]. The exposome [42, 43] comprises of all environmental exposures throughout the lifetime of an individual including individual-level exposures that arise from endogenous and exogenous activities (e.g., smoking, radiation, diet, physical activity, infectious agents, psychosocial stress, microbiome, medications, illicit drugs, cosmetics) and population level exposures (e.g., climate, air quality, urban environment, social capital) [42]. Exposure to individual chemicals, natural toxins, metals, uremic toxins (organic waste products that are excreted by the healthy kidney but accumulate and contribute to uremia in patients with CKD and generated in part by gut microbiome metabolism [44], and combination of these exposures throughout the lifespan contribute to kidney damage and kidney disease. Environmental exposure results in biological responses that include physiological alterations, metabolic changes, protein modifications, DNA mutations and adducts, epigenetic alterations, and perturbations of the microbiome [42]. Similar to GWAS and mGWAS studies, Exposome-Wide Association Study (EWAS) has been suggested [45] to discover association between exposures, the genome, and traits and diseases of interest by using high throughput data analytics methods.

Recent Findings in CKD Research

Untargeted and targeted metabolomics studies have been conducted using biospecimens obtained from clinical and epidemiological cohorts, as well as from in vivo and in vitro model systems to discover potential candidate biomarkers and mechanisms of CKD. The following section highlights some selected studies on CKD.

Systems Biology Approach (Phenotypic, Metabolomic, and Genetic Data) for Biomarker Discovery in CKD

Systems biology approach includes the integrated analysis of multi-omics data including genotypic, metabolic, and phenotypic data (Fig. 3.1). A mGWAS study conducted by Raffler et al. [46] identified and replicated 22 loci that had significant associations with urinary traits determined by targeted and non-targeted 1H NMR analysis of urine samples from 3861 participants of the SHIP-0 cohort and 1691 subjects of the KORA F4 cohort (for the follow-up), The authors reported that 15 of the loci were not reported in previous studies (HIBCH, CPS1, AGXT, XYLB, TKT, ETNPPL, SLC6A19, DMGDH, SLC36A2, GLDC, SLC6A13, ACSM3, SLC5A11,

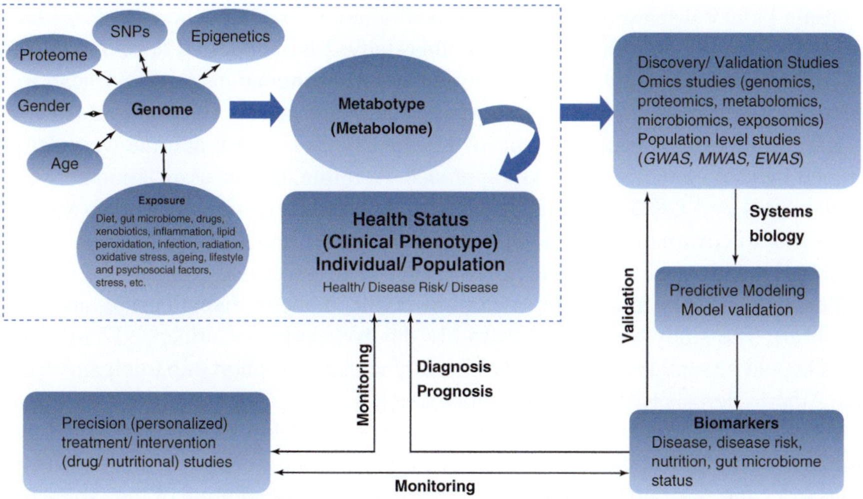

Fig. 3.1 Systems biology approaches to identify biomarkers for disease risk, stage of disease, disease treatment, or to mitigate against the development or progression of disease. The metabotype is a result of interactions of an individual's genes and environment throughout their lifetime. For a comprehensive study on biomarkers, study design should include metabotype, clinical phenotype(s), appropriate population cohorts, generation of multi-omics data, and data analytics methods. Discovered predictive biomarkers should be confirmed or validated within our across clinical or epidemiological cohorts using quantitative targeted analysis. Such biomarkers can be used for diagnosis and prognosis of disease risks, as well as for monitoring therapeutic or nutritional interventions

PNMT, SLC13A3). Two-thirds of the urinary loci also had a metabolite association in blood (reported in an earlier study). Significant associations were found to target the same metabolites in both urine and blood in six of these loci (CPS1 (glycine), AGXT2 (3-aminoisobutyrate), DMGDH (N,N-dimethylglycine), SLC6A13 (3-aminoisobutyrate), HPD (2-hydroxyisobutyrate), SLC5A11 (myo-inositol)). Directionality of the observed effect (an increase in metabolite concentration per copy of the effect allele), was found to be the same in both serum and urine for 5 of these 6 loci, whereas for SLC5A11 (associated with myo-inositol) showed opposite direction (an increase in urinary metabolite concentration per copy of the effect allele, as opposed to decreased levels reported in blood). These findings provide novel understandings into the relationship between homeostasis in blood and its regulation through excretion in urine. Furthermore, some of these newly discovered loci included genetic variants that were previously linked with CKD (CPS1, SLC6A13), pulmonary hypertension (CPS1), and ischemic stroke (XYLB). This study shows how genotype, metabotype, and phenotype can be connected to generate novel hypotheses about molecular mechanisms involved in the etiology of diseases.

Using a systems biology approach, McMohan and coworkers [47] investigated the association between urinary metabolites, genetic variants, and incident of chronic kidney disease (CKD) in the Framingham Offspring cohort to reveal biomarkers for early detection of CKD. In this study, 193 individuals developed CKD (eGFR under 60 ml/min/1.73 m^2) between cohort examinations 6 and 8 (mean follow-up of 9.7 years); which were age- and sex-matched to 193 controls (free of CKD). In this study, concentrations of 154 metabolites in fasting urine were determined by using a targeted LC-MS approach. Additionally, the association between metabolites and CKD was examined using logistic regression (with and without adjusting to covariates). The authors reported that increased levels of urinary glycine and histidine were found to be associated with lower risk of incident for CKD (after multivariable adjustment to baseline eGFR, diabetes, hypertension, and proteinuria). The study also found that only the association of urinary glycine with CKD could be replicated in a follow-up study with a sub cohort of participants from the Atherosclerosis Risk in Communities (ARIC) cohort. The authors further examined associations of these two metabolites with exome chip variants and found that the lead SNPs in association with glycine and histidine were to be rs77010315 in *SLC36A2* and rs35690712 in *SLC39A7*, respectively. The addition of these metabolites into the algorithm has led to a 4% discrimination improvement relative to the clinical model alone. Although these genes had links to solute transporters, none of these SNPs (rs77010315 and rs35690712) showed associations with eGFR/CKD [48] in the larger CKDGen exome chip dataset. Investigating associations of all metabolites with exome chip variant data found that 36 SNPs at 30 loci were significantly associated with 31 metabolites. Two of those metabolites, aminoisobutyric acid (urinary and serum) and nonanoylcarnitine (serum) were found to be associated with rs37370 in AGXT2 and rs2286963 in ACADL (and in hepatic mRNA), respectively, in previous mGWAS) studies [49, 50]. Furthermore, these significant exome chip findings were searched for associations of known renal phenotypes by looking for overlaps with known eGFR/CKD genes. It was found that intergenic region near SLC7A9 (rs8101881) was associated with increased urinary lysine and NG-monomethyl-L-arginine (NMMA) levels. The association of this SNP (rs8101881) could be confirmed in the CKDGen GWAS dataset in a direction-consistent manner. SLC7A9 is a gene that encodes a part of a transporter in the kidney that is responsible for reabsorbing positively charged amino acids from the urine including arginine, cystine, ornithine, and lysine [46]. In addition, NMMA is an arginine metabolite that is a known substrate for members of the SLC7 family of transporters. In this study, authors demonstrated that (a) low urinary glycine and histidine levels were associated with higher risk in incident CKD, (b) genomic association of urinary metabolomics discovered lysine and NMMA as being linked with CKD and provided further evidence for the association of SLC7A9 [51] with CKD. Thus, the study shows the importance of a systems biology approach (by combining phenotypic, metabolomic, and genetic data) for finding biomarkers of CKD. In addition, these findings merit further exploring perturbations in metabolic pathways (e.g., glycine is a metabolite involved in one carbon metabolism) where specific nutrients may be revealed that could aid in development of improved treatment strategies [52].

Arginine and Taurine as Biomarkers of Diabetic Nephropathy (DN)

Type 2 diabetes mellitus (T2DM) is a prominent cause of CKD because DN is a major complication in T2DM. In addition, DN is the leading cause of kidney disease in patients starting renal replacement therapy [3]. DN is generally defined based on the increased urinary albumin excretion (UAE) in the absence of other renal diseases and DN is categorized into stages based on UAE values: microalbuminuria (UAE ≥20 μg/min and ≤199 μg/min) and macroalbuminuria (UAE ≥200 μg/min). Increased high blood glucose (hyperglycemia), increased blood pressure levels, and genetic predisposition are considered to be the main risk factors for the development of DN [3]. Tao et al. [53] have evaluated serum metabolome in patients with biopsy proven DN (estimated GFR (eGFR) >60 mL $min^{-1}/1.73\ m^2$ and urine albumin creatinine ratio (UACR) ≥30 mg g^{-1}), age/ gender matched T2DM without renal diseases (T2DM, UACR <30 mg g^{-1}, and eGFR >60 mL $min^{-1}/1.73\ m^2$), age/ gender matched healthy controls (CTRL), and household contacts who were on the same diet of each patient on DM group (HH) by using untargeted LC-MS. The goals of their study were to explore differences in serum metabolic profiles between biopsy proven DN and T2DM, and to assess potential impact of diets and lifestyles on serum metabolome. A total of 1470 metabolites were identified in all serum samples and 45 metabolites were found with significantly different intensities between DN and DM (e.g., biliverdin and taurine were reduced while L-arginine was increased in DN comparing to DM). In this study, DN could be distinguished from age/gender matched DM patients without DN by serum L-arginine (AUC = 0.824) or taurine levels (AUC = 0.789) while L-Methionine, deethylatrazine, L-tryptophan and fumaric acid were reduced in DM comparing with those of CTRL group, and there was no differentiation found between DM and HH groups.

Influence of Microbiome in CKD

Emerging evidence suggests that the gut microbiome serves an important role in the development and progression of CKD. Dysbiosis in the gut microbiome can result in the generation of uraemic toxins in blood, increase in transportation of gut microbiome derived products into blood including lipopolysaccharides (LPS) (LPS initiate a signaling cascade that leads to proinflammatory gene activation), and it can lead to CKD [54, 55]. There are several published studies which investigate the association between the gut microbiome, uremic toxins, and CKD using biospecimens from humans and from animal models. Sun et al. [56] conducted a two-phase case-control study in a community health program to investigate the clinical association between metabolites and CKD using LC. The first phase included metabolomics analysis (UPLC-Q-TOF-MS) of biospecimens from participants collected at baseline and collected at the 1-year follow-up in a prospective case-control study.

The investigations focused on serum samples from individuals who showed a rapid decline of eGFR (eGFRRD) in yearly (eGFR decline >20%) compared to control group (yearly eGFR decline <5%). The authors indicated that 53 metabolites were identified and the intensity of histidine, indole-3-propionic acid (IPA), and paraxanthine were found to be significantly different between the eGFRRD and control groups. In addition, IPA was found to be different in the eGFRRD group at baseline. In the second phase, indoxyl sulfate and p-cresol sulfate levels were measured in samples from healthy subjects (n = 144) and CKD patients (n = 140) and average level of indoxyl sulfate and p-cresol sulfate were found to be significantly higher in the CKD patients, while the average level of IPA was significantly higher in the control patients indicating that IPA has a protective role in CKD. Indoxyl-3-sulfate and indole-3-propionic acids are microbial co-metabolites of tryptophan degradation [57] while p-cresol sulfate is a generated because of microbial degradation of tyrosine [58].

To elucidate the influence of microbiota to the retention of uremic solutes in CKD, Mishima et al. [59] analyzed biospecimens (capillary electrophoresis, CE-TOF-MS) from an adenine-induced renal failure mouse model, control mice under germ-free or specific pathogen-free (SPF) conditions. Mice with renal failure under germ-free conditions showed significant increase or decrease in plasma metabolites. Plasma levels of 11 major uremic toxins, were shown to be significantly lower in germ-free mice than in SPF mice with renal failure. These 11 metabolites are considered microbiota-derived uremic solutes that included indoxyl sulfate, p-cresyl sulfate, phenyl sulfate, cholate, hippurate, dimethylglycine, γ-guanidinobutyrate, glutarate, 2-hydroxypentanoate, trimethylamine N-oxide, and phenaceturate. These metabolites could be classified to three groups based on their origin: completely derived from microbiota (indoxyl sulfate, p-cresyl sulfate), derived from both host and microbiota (dimethylglycine), and derived from both microbiota and dietary components (trimethylamine N-oxide, (TMAO)). In addition, renal failure under germ-free conditions caused disappearance of fecal short-chain fatty acids, decreased utilization of intestinal amino acids, and severe kidney damage compared with SPF mice with renal failure indicating that microbiota-derived short-chain fatty acids and efficient amino acid utilization may have a protective effect on kidney, and loss of these factors may worsen renal damage in germ-free mice with renal failure. This study demonstrated that the gut microbiome can significantly contribute to generating harmful uremic solutes and, however, the absence of the microbiota can also have harmful effects on CKD progression.

TMAO, another uremic toxin, is a metabolite generated through gut microbiome related metabolism [60] [also endogenously biosynthesized from trimethylamine, which is derived from choline, which can be derived from dietary lecithin (phosphatidylcholines) or dietary carnitine] and it is linked with CKD. Missailidis et al. [25] measured trimethylamine-N-oxide (TMAO) and related metabolites (choline and betaine), using LC-MS/MS method, and assessed circulating levels of albumin, creatinine, calcium, phosphatase, hemoglobin, fibrinogen, and hsCRP), IL-6, and GFR in fasting plasma samples from 80 controls and 179 CKD stage 3–5 patients. Comorbidities and nutritional status of patients were assessed based on medical records, and subjective global assessment (SGA) score was used as a surrogate marker of protein-energy wasting (PEW). In this study, GFR was experimentally determined (mGFR) by Iohexol clearance in controls and CKD 3–4 patients. In CKD 5 patients (mGFR was calculated by the mean of renal urea and creatinine clearance from a 24-hour urine collection). eGFR used in follow-up after renal replacement therapy (Rtx) was calculated by a cystatin C-based equation for estimation of GFR. GFR was found to be the dominant variable affecting plasma TMAO, choline, and betaine levels. A longitudinal study (conducted for 5 years) of 74 CKD stage 5 patients starting renal transplant demonstrated that although dialysis treatment did not affect TMAO, Rtx reduced levels of TMAO to that of controls. Choline and betaine levels continued to increase following Rtx. In CKD 3–5 patients, TMAO levels were found to be associated with IL-6, fibrinogen (Rho = 0.43; $p < 0.0001$) and hsCRP. Furthermore, higher TMAO levels were found to be associated with an increased risk for all-cause mortality that remained significant after multivariate adjustment. This study shows that (a) elevated TMAO levels were strongly associated with degree of renal function in CKD and these levels normalize after renal transplantation, (b) TMAO levels correlate with increased systemic inflammation in CKD, (c) TMAO is an independent predictor of mortality in CKD 3–5 patients.

Precision Nutrition in Treatment and Prevention of CKD

Dietary and nutritional intervention is beneficial for managing CKD. Metabolic individuality or metabolic heterogeneity in humans that arises from differences in genetics, epigenetics, microbiome, lifestyle, dietary intake, and environmental exposure [61, 62] is believed to be responsible for variability in disease etiology, and the response to treatments and interventions. Thus, one size-fits-for-all concepts are no longer valid for treatment or intervention to CKD (as for other diseases), because of different severities, stages, and types of the kidney disease [63]. Therefore, precision nutrition-based approaches are needed for nutritional management of CKD in patients, including personalized treatment goals for different patients (Fig. 3.2) [63]. For example, dysbiosis of microbiome may be responsible for generating uremic toxins. Therefore, different dietary patterns such as more plant-based foods together with personalized consumption of prebiotics, probiotics, and synbiotics (mixture of prebiotics and probiotics) may beneficially alter the microbiota in CKD patients [44, 54, 64].

In a pilot study, Saggi et al. [66] performed a metabolomics analysis using baseline plasma samples obtained from patients previously diagnosed with CKD Stages III-IV who had participated in a dose escalation study that involved the probiotic Renadyl™. The goal of their study was to identify metabolites (and potential metabolic pathways involved) in baseline samples that differentiated patients with CKD whose blood urea nitrogen (BUN) decreased from those who had increased or experienced no change in BUN after using the probiotic for 4 months (increase in BUN was an indicative of progression of CKD). Results of univariate and multivariate

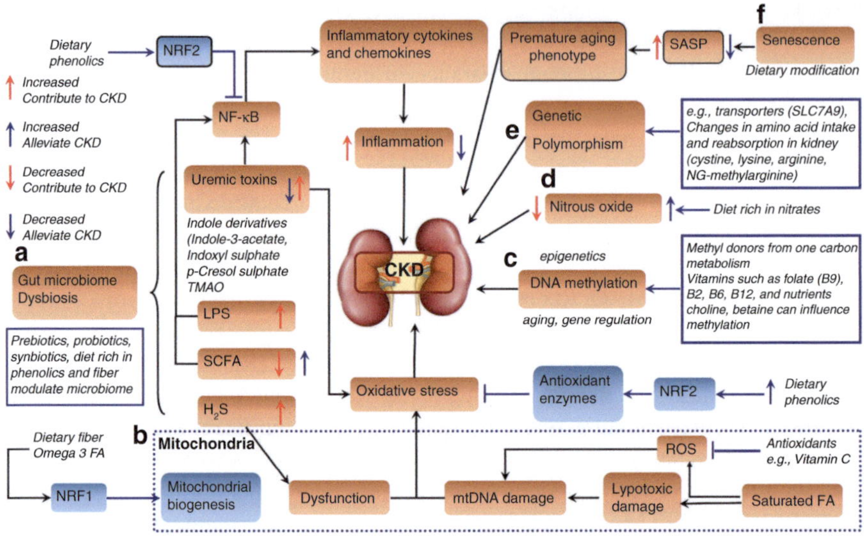

Fig. 3.2 Potential targets for nutritional (or dietary) intervention to mitigate against CKD progression. These nutritional or dietary interventions need to be personalized (for individuals or groups of individuals (with similar metabotype) to address variation in responses related to genetic polymorphisms. (**a**) Dysbiosis (imbalance) of gut microbiome can result from exposures, including unhealthy dietary habits. There is a bidirectional cause-effect that exists between gut microbiome dysbiosis and CKD. The dysbiosis generates uremic toxins, lowers short-chain fatty acids (SCFA), increases gut permeability, and increases bacterial lipopolysaccharides (LPS) in blood, increases toxins such as H_2S. These products lead to mitochondrial dysfunction, oxidative stress, and inflammation in CKD. Dietary modulation of gut microbiome can have many beneficial effects on alleviating CKD. (**b**) Saturated fats can generate reactive oxygen species (ROS), which cause mitochondrial DNA (mtDNA) damage leading to oxidative stress. Dietary phenolics upregulate nuclear factor erythroid 2-related factor 2 (NRF2) attenuating oxidative stress while SCFA reduces inflammation. (**c**) DNA methylation is an epigenetics mechanism that regulates gene expression, and epigenetics alterations may explain differences in gene expression in CKD such as oxidative stress, altered aging processes (reduced methylation etc.). (**d**) Oral bacteria convert nitrates (NO_3^-) in the diet into nitrites (NO_2^-) in mouth, NO_2^- enters the bloodstream, is converted into NO. NO promotes vasodilation and reduces blood pressure, inflammation, and oxidative stress benefiting CKD patients. Reduction in NO formation results in poor health outcomes in CKD. Consumption of food rich in nitrate is beneficial for CKD and cardiovascular diseases. (**e**) Genetic variants (SNPs) can perturb the expression and function of enzymes, transporters, or receptors and their ligands. Understanding these SNPs enables identifying responders or non-responders and to determine how much nutrient is needed for an individual or a group of individuals in interventions in CKD. (**f**) CKD is associated with various factors including those that lead to apoptosis resistance and the accumulation of senescent cells with a characteristic senescence-associated secretory phenotype (SASP). SARP leads to NF-KB and other inflammatory mediators triggering premature aging phenotype. Consumption of red meat (especially processed) and increased levels of uraemic toxins are among the factors that contribute to senescence and premature aging. Therefore, dietary modifications may delay premature aging in CKD. Sources: Mafra et al. [64], Zeisel [61], and Dodson et al. [65]

statistics analysis revealed metabolites that best differentiated these phenotypic groups. The sixteen patients who had a decrease in BUN were not significantly different based on demographic and clinical measures from those whose BUN increased or did not change except for age. Most of the metabolites that differentiated these phenotypic groups are known to be modulated by gut microflora, which may eventually provide a mechanistic link between probiotic and outcomes. This metabolomics analysis revealed metabolites at baseline that may predict individuals with CKD that would most benefit from a probiotics [66]. Additional examples for using food as medicine for targeting dysbiosis in microbiome, epigenetics alterations, senescence, mitochondrial dysfunction, and other perturbations in pathways in CKD are well reviewed in Mafra et al. [64].

Cupisti et al. [67], conducted and reported a case-control study to assess the effects of a pragmatic, stepwise, personalized nutritional support in the management of CKD patients (stages 3b-5 not-on-dialysis) on tertiary care. The Nutritional Treatment Group (NTG) in the study consisted of 305 patients (190 males, aged 70 ± 12 years) who received nutritional support while the control group (CG) consisted of 518 patients (281 males, aged 73 ± 13 years) who did not receive any dietary therapy. In the NTG, the dietary interventions were assigned to prevent or to correct abnormalities and to maintain a good nutritional status. These interventions included manipulation of sodium, phosphate, energy, and protein dietary intakes while paying special attention to each patient's dietary habits. Clinical and biochemical data in the study were extracted from the medical records and routine lab methods were used to obtain biochemistry data. In this study, lover levels of phosphate and blood urea nitrogen (BUN) were found to be lower in the NTG than in the CG, especially in stage 4 and 5. The occurrence of hyperphosphatemia (high phosphate levels in blood) was found to be significantly lower in the NTG than in CG in stage 5 ($p < 0.001$), in stage 4 ($p < 0.001$) and stage 3b ($p < 0.05$). In addition, serum albumin was found to be higher in NTG than in CG especially in stage 5. Furthermore, the use of calcium-free intestinal phosphate binders was found to be significantly lower in NTG than in CG ($p < 0.01$), as well as that of Erythropoiesis stimulating agents ($p < 0.01$), and active Vitamin D preparations ($p <0.01$). This study showed the usefulness of a nutritional support in addition to the pharmacological good practice in CKD patients on tertiary care to deliver preferable outcomes: Lowering phosphate and BUN levels together with maintenance of serum albumin levels, a lower need of erythropoiesis stimulating agents, phosphate binders and active Vitamin D preparations in NTG). This study highlights the usefulness of personalized nutrition approach in the management of the CKD patients.

Concluding Remarks

CKD is a major cause of mortality worldwide. Most often CKD is diagnosed when it is in the advanced stages of the disease. There is a need to understand both genetic and non-genetic drivers of CKD to improve diagnose, especially early on, and to reveal mechanisms of disease and progression. Advances in omics-based methodologies, together with advancing data analytic techniques, have provided the tools for identifying biomarkers to diagnose stages of CKD, monitor therapeutic and nutritional interventions, and derive new interventions. Treatment or nutritional intervention for CKD (and many other diseases) needs to be personalized due to metabolic individuality or heterogeneity between individuals in populations as shown by GWAS, mGWAS, and other studies.

References

1. Chen TK, Knicely DH, Grams ME. Chronic kidney disease diagnosis and management: a review. JAMA. 2019;322(13):1294–304. https://doi.org/10.1001/jama.2019.14745.
2. Neuen BL, Chadban SJ, Demaio AR, Johnson DW, Perkovic V. Chronic kidney disease and the global NCDs agenda. BMJ Glob Health. 2017;2(2):e000380. https://doi.org/10.1136/bmjgh-2017-000380.
3. Gross J, de Azevedo M, Silveiro SP, Canani LI, Caramori ML, Zelmanovitz T. Diabetic nephropathy diagnosis, prevention, and treatment. Diabetes Care. 2005;28(1):164–76.
4. Webster AC, Nagler EV, Morton RL, Masson P. Chronic kidney disease. Lancet. 2017;389(10075):1238–52. https://doi.org/10.1016/s0140-6736(16)32064-5.
5. Delanaye P, Mariat C. The applicability of eGFR equations to different populations. Nat Rev Nephrol. 2013;9(9):513–22. https://doi.org/10.1038/nrneph.2013.143.
6. Romagnani P, Remuzzi G, Glassock R, Levin A, Jager KJ, Tonelli M, Massy Z, Wanner C, Anders HJ. Chronic kidney disease. Nat Rev Dis Primers. 2017;3:17088. https://doi.org/10.1038/nrdp.2017.88.
7. Mounicou S, Szpunar J, Lobinski R. Metallomics: the concept and methodology. Chem Soc Rev. 2009;38(4):1119–38. https://doi.org/10.1039/b713633c.
8. Dupre TV, Schnellmann RG, Miller GW. Using the exposome to address gene-environment interactions in kidney disease. Nat Rev Nephrol. 2020;16(11):621–2. https://doi.org/10.1038/s41581-020-0302-9.
9. Hocher B, Adamski J. Metabolomics for clinical use and research in chronic kidney disease. Nat Rev Nephrol. 2017;13(5):269–84. https://doi.org/10.1038/nrneph.2017.30.
10. Mendez KM, Reinke SN, Broadhurst DI. A comparative evaluation of the generalised predictive ability of eight machine learning algorithms across ten clinical metabolomics data sets for binary classification. Metabolomics. 2019;15(12):150. https://doi.org/10.1007/s11306-019-1612-4.
11. Ren S, Hinzman AA, Kang EL, Szczesniak RD, Lu LJ. Computational and statistical analysis of metabolomics data. Metabolomics. 2015;11(6):1492–513. https://doi.org/10.1007/s11306-015-0823-6.
12. Trygg J, Holmes E, Lundstedt T. Chemometrics in metabonomics. J Proteome Res. 2007;6:469–79.
13. Sumner SCJ, McRitchie S, Pathmasiri W. Metabolomics for biomarker discovery and to derive genetic links to disease. In: Caterina RD, Martinez JA, Kohlmeier M, editors. Principles of nutrigenetics and nutrigenomics. Cambridge: Academic; 2020. p. 75–9.
14. Johnson CH, Gonzalez FJ. Challenges and opportunities of metabolomics. J Cell Physiol. 2012;227(8):2975–81. https://doi.org/10.1002/jcp.24002.
15. Everett JR, Holmes E, Veselkov KA, Lindon JC, Nicholson JK. A unified conceptual framework for metabolic phenotyping in diagnosis and prognosis. Trends Pharmacol Sci. 2019;40(10):763–73. https://doi.org/10.1016/j.tips.2019.08.004.

16. Nicholson JK, Holmes E, Kinross JM, Darzi AW, Takats Z, Lindon JC. Metabolic phenotyping in clinical and surgical environments. Nature. 2012;491(7424):384–92. https://doi.org/10.1038/nature11708.
17. Johnson CH, Patterson AD, Idle JR, Gonzalez FJ. Xenobiotic metabolomics: major impact on the metabolome. Annu Rev Pharmacol Toxicol. 2012;52:37–56. https://doi.org/10.1146/annurev-pharmtox-010611-134748.
18. Stewart DA, Dhungana S, Clark RF, Pathmasiri WW, McRitchie SL, Sumner SJ. Omics technologies used in systems biology. In: Fry R, editor. Systems biology in toxicology and environmental health. 1st ed. Waltham: Academic; 2015. p. 57–84.
19. Sumner SCJ, Pathmasiri W, Carlson JE, McRitchie SL, Fennell TR. Metabolomics. In: Smart R, Hodgeson E, editors. Molecular and biochemical toxicology. 5th ed. Hoboken: Wiley; 2018. p. 115–31.
20. Ryan D, Robards K. Metabolomics: the greatest omics of them all? Trends Anal Chem. 2005;24:285–93.
21. Holmes E, Wilson ID, Nicholson JK. Metabolic phenotyping in health and disease. Cell. 2008;134(5):714–7. https://doi.org/10.1016/j.cell.2008.08.026.
22. Robinette SL, Lindon JC, Nicholson JK. Statistical spectroscopic tools for biomarker discovery and systems medicine. Anal Chem. 2013;85(11):5297–303. https://doi.org/10.1021/ac4007254.
23. Brennan L. Use of metabotyping for optimal nutrition. Curr Opin Biotechnol. 2017;44:35–8. https://doi.org/10.1016/j.copbio.2016.10.008.
24. Roberts LD, Souza AL, Gerszten RE, Clish CB. Targeted metabolomics. Curr Protoc Mol Biol. 2012;32:31–24. https://doi.org/10.1002/0471142727.mb3002s98.
25. Missailidis C, Hallqvist J, Qureshi AR, Barany P, Heimburger O, Lindholm B, Stenvinkel P, Bergman P. Serum trimethylamine-N-oxide is strongly related to renal function and predicts outcome in chronic kidney disease. PLoS One. 2016;11(1):e0141738. https://doi.org/10.1371/journal.pone.0141738.
26. Duranton F, Lundin U, Gayrard N, Mischak H, Aparicio M, Mourad G, Daures JP, Weinberger KM, Argiles A. Plasma and urinary amino acid metabolomic profiling in patients with different levels of kidney function. Clin J Am Soc Nephrol. 2014;9(1):37–45. https://doi.org/10.2215/CJN.06000613.
27. Bird SS, Sheldon DP, Gathungu RM, Vouros P, Kautz R, Matson WR, Kristal BS. Structural characterization of plasma metabolites detected via LC-electrochemical coulometric array using LC-UV fractionation, MS, and NMR. Anal Chem. 2012;84(22):9889–98. https://doi.org/10.1021/ac302278u.
28. Sasaki K, Sagawa H, Suzuki M, Yamamoto H, Tomita M, Soga T, Ohashi Y. A metabolomics platform by capillary electrophoresis coupled with a high-resolution mass spectrometry for plasma analysis. Anal Chem. 2018;91(2):1295–301. https://doi.org/10.1021/acs.analchem.8b02994.
29. Pathmasiri W, Kay K, McRitchie S, Sumner S. Analysis of NMR metabolomics data. Methods Mol Biol. 2020;2104:61–97. https://doi.org/10.1007/978-1-0716-0239-3_5.
30. Fan TW, Lane AN. NMR-based stable isotope resolved metabolomics in systems biochemistry. J Biomol NMR. 2011;49(3-4):267–80. https://doi.org/10.1007/s10858-011-9484-6.
31. Bictash M, Ebbels TM, Chan Q, Loo RL, Yap IK, Brown IJ, de Iorio M, Daviglus ML, Holmes E, Stamler J, Nicholson JK, Elliott P. Opening up the "Black Box": metabolic phenotyping and metabolome-wide association studies in epidemiology. J Clin Epidemiol. 2010;63(9):970–9. https://doi.org/10.1016/j.jclinepi.2009.10.001.
32. Hedjazi L, Gauguier D, Zalloua PA, Nicholson JK, Dumas ME, Cazier JB. mQTL.NMR: an integrated suite for genetic mapping of quantitative variations of (1)H NMR-based metabolic profiles. Anal Chem. 2015;87(8):4377–84. https://doi.org/10.1021/acs.analchem.5b00145.
33. Cazier JB, Kaisaki PJ, Argoud K, Blaise BJ, Veselkov K, Ebbels TM, Tsang T, Wang Y, Bihoreau MT, Mitchell SC, Holmes EC, Lindon JC, Scott J, Nicholson JK, Dumas ME, Gauguier D. Untargeted metabolome quantitative trait locus mapping associates variation in

urine glycerate to mutant glycerate kinase. J Proteome Res. 2012;11(2):631–42. https://doi.org/10.1021/pr200566t.

34. Sekula P, Goek ON, Quaye L, Barrios C, Levey AS, Romisch-Margl W, Menni C, Yet I, Gieger C, Inker LA, Adamski J, Gronwald W, Illig T, Dettmer K, Krumsiek J, Oefner PJ, Valdes AM, Meisinger C, Coresh J, Spector TD, Mohney RP, Suhre K, Kastenmuller G, Kottgen A. A metabolome-wide association study of kidney function and disease in the general population. J Am Soc Nephrol. 2016;27(4):1175–88. https://doi.org/10.1681/ASN.2014111099.
35. Kraus WE, Muoio DM, Stevens R, Craig D, Bain JR, Grass E, Haynes C, Kwee L, Qin X, Slentz DH, Krupp D, Muehlbauer M, Hauser ER, Gregory SG, Newgard CB, Shah SH. Metabolomic quantitative trait loci (mQTL) mapping implicates the ubiquitin proteasome system in cardiovascular disease pathogenesis. PLoS Genet. 2015;11(11):e1005553. https://doi.org/10.1371/journal.pgen.1005553.
36. Gieger C, Geistlinger L, Altmaier E, Hrabe de Angelis M, Kronenberg F, Meitinger T, Mewes HW, Wichmann HE, Weinberger KM, Adamski J, Illig T, Suhre K. Genetics meets metabolomics: a genome-wide association study of metabolite profiles in human serum. PLoS Genet. 2008;4(11):e1000282. https://doi.org/10.1371/journal.pgen.1000282.
37. Gurdasani D, Barroso I, Zeggini E, Sandhu MS. Genomics of disease risk in globally diverse populations. Nat Rev Genet. 2019;20(9):520–35. https://doi.org/10.1038/s41576-019-0144-0.
38. Sandholm N, McKnight AJ, Salem RM, Brennan EP, Forsblom C, Harjutsalo V, Makinen VP, McKay GJ, Sadlier DM, Williams WW, Martin F, Panduru NM, Tarnow L, Tuomilehto J, Tryggvason K, Zerbini G, Comeau ME, Langefeld CD, Consortium F, Godson C, Hirschhorn JN, Maxwell AP, Florez JC, Groop PH, FinnDiane Study G, the GC. Chromosome 2q31.1 associates with ESRD in women with type 1 diabetes. J Am Soc Nephrol. 2013;24(10):1537–43. https://doi.org/10.1681/ASN.2012111122.
39. Kottgen A, Glazer NL, Dehghan A, Hwang SJ, Katz R, Li M, Yang Q, Gudnason V, Launer LJ, Harris TB, Smith AV, Arking DE, Astor BC, Boerwinkle E, Ehret GB, Ruczinski I, Scharpf RB, Chen YD, de Boer IH, Haritunians T, Lumley T, Sarnak M, Siscovick D, Benjamin EJ, Levy D, Upadhyay A, Aulchenko YS, Hofman A, Rivadeneira F, Uitterlinden AG, van Duijn CM, Chasman DI, Pare G, Ridker PM, Kao WH, Witteman JC, Coresh J, Shlipak MG, Fox CS. Multiple loci associated with indices of renal function and chronic kidney disease. Nat Genet. 2009;41(6):712–7. https://doi.org/10.1038/ng.377.
40. Wild CP. Complementing the genome with an "exposome": the outstanding challenge of environmental exposure measurement in molecular epidemiology. Cancer Epidemiol Biomark Prev. 2005;14(8):1847–50. https://doi.org/10.1158/1055-9965.EPI-05-0456.
41. Wild CP. The exposome: from concept to utility. Int J Epidemiol. 2012;41(1):24–32. https://doi.org/10.1093/ije/dyr236.
42. Niedzwiecki MM, Walker DI, Vermeulen R, Chadeau-Hyam M, Jones DP, Miller GW. The exposome: molecules to populations. Annu Rev Pharmacol Toxicol. 2019;59:107–27. https://doi.org/10.1146/annurev-pharmtox-010818-021315.
43. Rappaport SM, Barupal DK, Wishart D, Vineis P, Scalbert A. The blood exposome and its role in discovering causes of disease. Environ Health Perspect. 2014;122(8):769–74. https://doi.org/10.1289/ehp.1308015.
44. Vitetta L, Gobe G. Uremia and chronic kidney disease: the role of the gut microflora and therapies with pro- and prebiotics. Mol Nutr Food Res. 2013;57(5):824–32. https://doi.org/10.1002/mnfr.201200714.
45. Manrai AK, Cui Y, Bushel PR, Hall M, Karakitsios S, Mattingly CJ, Ritchie M, Schmitt C, Sarigiannis DA, Thomas DC, Wishart D, Balshaw DM, Patel CJ. Informatics and data analytics to support exposome-based discovery for public health. Annu Rev Public Health. 2017;38:279–94. https://doi.org/10.1146/annurev-publhealth-082516-012737.
46. Raffler J, Friedrich N, Arnold M, Kacprowski T, Rueedi R, Altmaier E, Bergmann S, Budde K, Gieger C, Homuth G, Pietzner M, Romisch-Margl W, Strauch K, Volzke H, Waldenberger M, Wallaschofski H, Nauck M, Volker U, Kastenmuller G, Suhre K. Genome-wide association study with targeted and non-targeted NMR metabolomics identifies 15 novel loci of urinary human metabolic individuality. PLoS Genet. 2015;11(9):e1005487. https://doi.org/10.1371/journal.pgen.1005487.

47. McMahon GM, Hwang S-J, Clish CB, Tin A, Yang Q, Larson MG, Rhee EP, Li M, Levy D, O'Donnell CJ. Urinary metabolites along with common and rare genetic variations are associated with incident chronic kidney disease. Kidney Int. 2017;91(6):1426–35.
48. Wuttke M, Li Y, Li M, Sieber KB, Feitosa MF, Gorski M, Tin A, Wang L, Chu AY, Hoppmann A, Kirsten H, Giri A, Chai JF, Sveinbjornsson G, Tayo BO, Nutile T, Fuchsberger C, Marten J, Cocca M, Ghasemi S, Xu Y, Horn K, Noce D, van der Most PJ, Sedaghat S, Yu Z, Akiyama M, Afaq S, Ahluwalia TS, Almgren P, Amin N, Arnlov J, Bakker SJL, Bansal N, Baptista D, Bergmann S, Biggs ML, Biino G, Boehnke M, Boerwinkle E, Boissel M, Bottinger EP, Boutin TS, Brenner H, Brumat M, Burkhardt R, Butterworth AS, Campana E, Campbell A, Campbell H, Canouil M, Carroll RJ, Catamo E, Chambers JC, Chee ML, Chee ML, Chen X, Cheng CY, Cheng Y, Christensen K, Cifkova R, Ciullo M, Concas MP, Cook JP, Coresh J, Corre T, Sala CF, Cusi D, Danesh J, Daw EW, de Borst MH, De Grandi A, de Mutsert R, de Vries APJ, Degenhardt F, Delgado G, Demirkan A, Di Angelantonio E, Dittrich K, Divers J, Dorajoo R, Eckardt KU, Ehret G, Elliott P, Endlich K, Evans MK, Felix JF, Foo VHX, Franco OH, Franke A, Freedman BI, Freitag-Wolf S, Friedlander Y, Froguel P, Gansevoort RT, Gao H, Gasparini P, Gaziano JM, Giedraitis V, Gieger C, Girotto G, Giulianini F, Gogele M, Gordon SD, Gudbjartsson DF, Gudnason V, Haller T, Hamet P, Harris TB, Hartman CA, Hayward C, Hellwege JN, Heng CK, Hicks AA, Hofer E, Huang W, Hutri-Kahonen N, Hwang SJ, Ikram MA, Indridason OS, Ingelsson E, Ising M, Jaddoe VWV, Jakobsdottir J, Jonas JB, Joshi PK, Josyula NS, Jung B, Kahonen M, Kamatani Y, Kammerer CM, Kanai M, Kastarinen M, Kerr SM, Khor CC, Kiess W, Kleber ME, Koenig W, Kooner JS, Korner A, Kovacs P, Kraja AT, Krajcoviechova A, Kramer H, Kramer BK, Kronenberg F, Kubo M, Kuhnel B, Kuokkanen M, Kuusisto J, La Bianca M, Laakso M, Lange LA, Langefeld CD, Lee JJ, Lehne B, Lehtimaki T, Lieb W, Lifelines Cohort S, Lim SC, Lind L, Lindgren CM, Liu J, Liu J, Loeffler M, Loos RJF, Lucae S, Lukas MA, Lyytikainen LP, Magi R, Magnusson PKE, Mahajan A, Martin NG, Martins J, Marz W, Mascalzoni D, Matsuda K, Meisinger C, Meitinger T, Melander O, Metspalu A, Mikaelsdottir EK, Milaneschi Y, Miliku K, Mishra PP, Program VAMV, Mohlke KL, Mononen N, Montgomery GW, Mook-Kanamori DO, Mychaleckyj JC, Nadkarni GN, Nalls MA, Nauck M, Nikus K, Ning B, Nolte IM, Noordam R, O'Connell J, O'Donoghue ML, Olafsson I, Oldehinkel AJ, Orho-Melander M, Ouwehand WH, Padmanabhan S, Palmer ND, Palsson R, Penninx B, Perls T, Perola M, Pirastu M, Pirastu N, Pistis G, Podgornaia AI, Polasek O, Ponte B, Porteous DJ, Poulain T, Pramstaller PP, Preuss MH, Prins BP, Province MA, Rabelink TJ, Raffield LM, Raitakari OT, Reilly DF, Rettig R, Rheinberger M, Rice KM, Ridker PM, Rivadeneira F, Rizzi F, Roberts DJ, Robino A, Rossing P, Rudan I, Rueedi R, Ruggiero D, Ryan KA, Saba Y, Sabanayagam C, Salomaa V, Salvi E, Saum KU, Schmidt H, Schmidt R, Schottker B, Schulz CA, Schupf N, Shaffer CM, Shi Y, Smith AV, Smith BH, Soranzo N, Spracklen CN, Strauch K, Stringham HM, Stumvoll M, Svensson PO, Szymczak S, Tai ES, Tajuddin SM, Tan NYQ, Taylor KD, Teren A, Tham YC, Thiery J, Thio CHL, Thomsen H, Thorleifsson G, Toniolo D, Tonjes A, Tremblay J, Tzoulaki I, Uitterlinden AG, Vaccargiu S, van Dam RM, van der Harst P, van Duijn CM, Velez Edward DR, Verweij N, Vogelezang S, Volker U, Vollenweider P, Waeber G, Waldenberger M, Wallentin L, Wang YX, Wang C, Waterworth DM, Bin Wei W, White H, Whitfield JB, Wild SH, Wilson JF, Wojczynski MK, Wong C, Wong TY, Xu L, Yang Q, Yasuda M, Yerges-Armstrong LM, Zhang W, Zonderman AB, Rotter JI, Bochud M, Psaty BM, Vitart V, Wilson JG, Dehghan A, Parsa A, Chasman DI, Ho K, Morris AP, Devuyst O, Akilesh S, Pendergrass SA, Sim X, Boger CA, Okada Y, Edwards TL, Snieder H, Stefansson K, Hung AM, Heid IM, Scholz M, Teumer A, Kottgen A, Pattaro C. A catalog of genetic loci associated with kidney function from analyses of a million individuals. Nat Genet. 2019;51(6):957–72. https://doi.org/10.1038/s41588-019-0407-x.
49. Illig T, Gieger C, Zhai G, Romisch-Margl W, Wang-Sattler R, Prehn C, Altmaier E, Kastenmuller G, Kato BS, Mewes HW, Meitinger T, de Angelis MH, Kronenberg F, Soranzo N, Wichmann HE, Spector TD, Adamski J, Suhre K. A genome-wide perspective of genetic variation in human metabolism. Nat Genet. 2010;42(2):137–41. https://doi.org/10.1038/ng.507.

50. Mirkov S, Myers JL, Ramirez J, Liu W. SNPs affecting serum metabolomic traits may regulate gene transcription and lipid accumulation in the liver. Metabolism. 2012;61(11):1523–7. https://doi.org/10.1016/j.metabol.2012.05.004.
51. Suhre K, Wallaschofski H, Raffler J, Friedrich N, Haring R, Michael K, Wasner C, Krebs A, Kronenberg F, Chang D, Meisinger C, Wichmann HE, Hoffmann W, Volzke H, Volker U, Teumer A, Biffar R, Kocher T, Felix SB, Illig T, Kroemer HK, Gieger C, Romisch-Margl W, Nauck M. A genome-wide association study of metabolic traits in human urine. Nat Genet. 2011;43(6):565–9. https://doi.org/10.1038/ng.837.
52. Ducker GS, Rabinowitz JD. One-carbon metabolism in health and disease. Cell Metab. 2017;25(1):27–42. https://doi.org/10.1016/j.cmet.2016.08.009.
53. Tao S, Zheng W, Liu Y, Li L, Li L, Ren Q, Shi M, Liu J, Jiang J, Ma H, Huang Z, Xia Z, Pan J, Wei T, Wang Y, Li P, Lan T, Ma L, Fu P. Analysis of serum metabolomics among biopsy-proven diabetic nephropathy, type 2 diabetes mellitus and healthy controls. RSC Adv. 2019;9(33):18713–9. https://doi.org/10.1039/c9ra01561b.
54. Esgalhado M, Kemp JA, Damasceno NR, Fouque D, Mafra D. Short-chain fatty acids a link between prebiotics and microbiota in chronic kidney disease. Future Microbiol. 2017;12(15):1413–25.
55. De Mauri A, Carrera D, Bagnati M, Rolla R, Chiarinotti D, Mogna L, Pane M, Amoruso A, Del Piano M. Probiotics-addicted low-protein diet for microbiota modulation in patients with advanced chronic kidney disease (ProLowCKD): a protocol of placebo-controlled randomized trial. J Funct Foods. 2020;74:104133. https://doi.org/10.1016/j.jff.2020.104133.
56. Sun CY, Lin CJ, Pan HC, Lee CC, Lu SC, Hsieh YT, Huang SY, Huang HY. Clinical association between the metabolite of healthy gut microbiota, 3-indolepropionic acid and chronic kidney disease. Clin Nutr. 2019;38(6):2945–8. https://doi.org/10.1016/j.clnu.2018.11.029.
57. Neves AL, Chilloux J, Sarafian MH, Rahim MB, Boulange CL, Dumas ME. The microbiome and its pharmacological targets: therapeutic avenues in cardiometabolic diseases. Curr Opin Pharmacol. 2015;25:36–44. https://doi.org/10.1016/j.coph.2015.09.013.
58. Viaene L, Thijs L, Jin Y, Liu Y, Gu Y, Meijers B, Claes K, Staessen J, Evenepoel P. Heritability and clinical determinants of serum indoxyl sulfate and p-cresyl sulfate, candidate biomarkers of the human microbiome enterotype. PLoS One. 2014;9(5):e79682. https://doi.org/10.1371/journal.pone.0079682.
59. Mishima E, Fukuda S, Mukawa C, Yuri A, Kanemitsu Y, Matsumoto Y, Akiyama Y, Fukuda NN, Tsukamoto H, Asaji K, Shima H, Kikuchi K, Suzuki C, Suzuki T, Tomioka Y, Soga T, Ito S, Abe T. Evaluation of the impact of gut microbiota on uremic solute accumulation by a CE-TOFMS-based metabolomics approach. Kidney Int. 2017;92(3):634–45. https://doi.org/10.1016/j.kint.2017.02.011.
60. Tang WH, Wang Z, Kennedy DJ, Wu Y, Buffa JA, Agatisa-Boyle B, Li XS, Levison BS, Hazen SL. Gut microbiota-dependent trimethylamine N-oxide (TMAO) pathway contributes to both development of renal insufficiency and mortality risk in chronic kidney disease. Circ Res. 2015;116(3):448–55. https://doi.org/10.1161/CIRCRESAHA.116.305360.
61. Zeisel SH. Precision (personalized) nutrition: understanding metabolic heterogeneity. Annu Rev Food Sci Technol. 2020;11:71–92. https://doi.org/10.1146/annurev-food-032519-051736.
62. Luttropp K, Lindholm B, Carrero JJ, Glorieux G, Schepers E, Vanholder R, Schalling M, Stenvinkel P, Nordfors L. Genetics/genomics in chronic kidney disease–towards personalized medicine? Semin Dial. 2009;22(4):417–22. https://doi.org/10.1111/j.1525-139X.2009.00592.x.
63. Kalantar-Zadeh K, Moore LW. Precision nutrition and personalized diet plan for kidney health and kidney disease management. J Ren Nutr. 2020;30(5):365–7. https://doi.org/10.1053/j.jrn.2020.07.005.
64. Mafra D, Borges NA, Lindholm B, Shiels PG, Evenepoel P, Stenvinkel P. Food as medicine: targeting the uraemic phenotype in chronic kidney disease. Nat Rev Nephrol. 2020;17(3):153–71. https://doi.org/10.1038/s41581-020-00345-8.

65. Dodson M, de la Vega MR, Cholanians AB, Schmidlin CJ, Chapman E, Zhang DD. Modulating NRF_2 in disease: timing is everything. Annu Rev Pharmacol Toxicol. 2019;59:555–75.
66. Saggi SJ, Mercier K, Gooding JR, Friedman E, Vyas U, Ranganathan N, Ranganathan P, McRitchie S, Sumner S. Metabolic profiling of a chronic kidney disease cohort reveals metabolic phenotype more likely to benefit from a probiotic. Int J Probiot Prebiot. 2017;12(1):43–54.
67. Cupisti A, D'Alessandro C, Di Iorio B, Bottai A, Zullo C, Giannese D, Barsotti M, Egidi MF. Nutritional support in the tertiary care of patients affected by chronic renal insufficiency: report of a step-wise, personalized, pragmatic approach. BMC Nephrol. 2016;17(1):124. https://doi.org/10.1186/s12882-016-0342-3.

Chapter 4
Microbiome Derived Metabolites in CKD and ESRD

Rohan Paul, Carolyn Feibig, and Dominic S. Raj

Introduction

Microbiota refers to the assemblage of microorganisms (composed of bacteria, archaea, bacteriophage, fungi, protozoa, and viruses) present in an environment. The microbiome is defined as the collective genomes of the microbes that live inside and on the human body. Host genetic factors affect microbial composition [1]. However, the microbial communities that are acquired postnatally by vertical transmission is continuously shaped by diet, medications, and other environmental exposures throughout life [2–4]. The Human Microbiome Project noted that the microbiome is unique for each individual, with each niche displaying one or a few signature taxa, and diversity is greatest in the gut with little variation over time [5]. Human gut harbors a complex community of over 100 trillion microbial cells, which constitute the gut microbiota [6]. The gut microbiome encodes about 3.3 million genes, which is 150 times more genes than our own genome [7]. The symbiotic gut microbiota provides complementary biological and metabolic functions that cannot be performed by humans [8].

R. Paul · D. S. Raj (✉)
Division of Kidney Diseases and Hypertension, Medical Facuty Associates - George Washington University, Washington, DC, USA

C. Feibig
INOVA Fairfax Hospital, Falls Church, VA, USA
e-mail: carolyn.feibig@inova.org

S. J. Saggi, M. O. Salifu (eds.), *Technological Advances in Care of Patients with Kidney Diseases*, https://doi.org/10.1007/978-3-031-11942-2_4

Microbiome in Health and Disease

The gut microbiome, comprising the collective genomes of the communities of commensal microbes (microbiota) that colonize the gut is involved in numerous physiological processes, including nutrient extraction/synthesis, metabolism, and immune regulation [9–12]. Gut dysbiosis is characterized frequently by decreased diversity, and also relative abundance of selected microbial taxa [13]. Pathological features of gut dysbiosis include generation of adverse metabolites, increased endotoxin release, augmentation of pro-inflammatory signals, and increased permeability to gut-derived molecules [14, 15]. Dysbiosis has been linked to a number of diseases such as obesity, diabetes, neurological diseases, colitis, kidney diseases, and CVD [16–23].

Microbiome in Kidney Disease

Altered gut microbial composition and function in renal insufficiency has been well characterized using cell culture, phylogenetic microarray, and 16S rDNA amplification. The reader is directed to the comprehensive review by Ramezani and colleagues for detailed account of the subject and techniques employed [24]. In an analysis of microbial DNA found in stool specimens among 24 individuals with ESRD and 12 healthy subjects, Vaziri and colleagues reported significant variation within 190 bacterial operational taxonomic units (OTUs)—namely *Brachybacterium*, *Catenibacterium*, *Enterobacteriaceae*, *Halomonadaceae*, *Moraxellaceae*, *Nesterenkonia*, *Polyangiaceae*, *Pseudomonadaceae*, and *Thiothrix* families that were increased in those with ESRD [25]. The investigators also demonstrated the putative role of uremia in driving this phenomenon using a rat model in which nephrectomized animals' stool cultures manifested variation in 175 OTUs from those that underwent sham surgery. A subsequent analysis by the same group found an overrepresentation of bacterial families carrying urease, uricase, and indole and p-cresol forming enzymes, and contraction of families with butyrate-forming enzymes [26]. The metabolic implications of these observations is discussed below. In a comparison between ESRD patients and healthy subjects, Hida and colleagues found lower quantities of *Bifidobacteria* and higher quantities of *Clostridium perfringens* through 16S rDNA amplification and DNA pyrosequencing [27]. Gao and colleagues examined the microbiome profile in peritoneal dialysis (PD) patients using metagenomic shotgun sequencing. The five most abundant phyla in decreasing order, were *Firmicutes*, *Bacteroidetes*, *Actinobacteria*, *Proteobacteria*, and *Verrucomicrobia* [28]. Surprisingly, the microbiome in PD patients was not significantly different from individuals without CKD.

Early alterations in gut microbiome in CKD is possibly adaptive, but becomes maladaptive with progressive loss of kidney function and contributes to uremic toxicity [29]. Dysbiosis in CKD may be a direct or indirect effect of uremia. For instance, urea secreted into the gastrointestinal tract in CKD is hydrolyzed by bacterial urease generating ammonia which alters the growth of commensal bacteria [30]. Other contributing indirect factors relevant to patients with kidney failure include decreased consumption of dietary fiber [31], frequent use of antibiotics [32], slow colonic transit [33], and potassium secretion by colon in advanced CKD [34].

Microbiome Derived Metabolites

The gastrointestinal system is at the interphase between the blood and the potentially toxic contents of the gut [35]. Uremia increases intestinal permeability, permitting translocation of bacteria and endotoxin across the intestinal wall [15, 36].

Colonic microbial fermentation of ingested proteins may lead to the formation of potentially toxic metabolites including ammonia, phenols, indoles, and amines (refer to Fig. 4.1) [37, 38]. This in concert with diminished generation of (inherently beneficial) short-chain fatty acids (SCFAs) compounded by gut epithelial hyperpermeability may lead to downstream consequences [14, 15, 26]. An understanding of these metabolites and their clinical significance in gut dysbiosis along with downstream consequences may reveal options for intervention and are reviewed here (refer to Table 4.1 and Fig. 4.2).

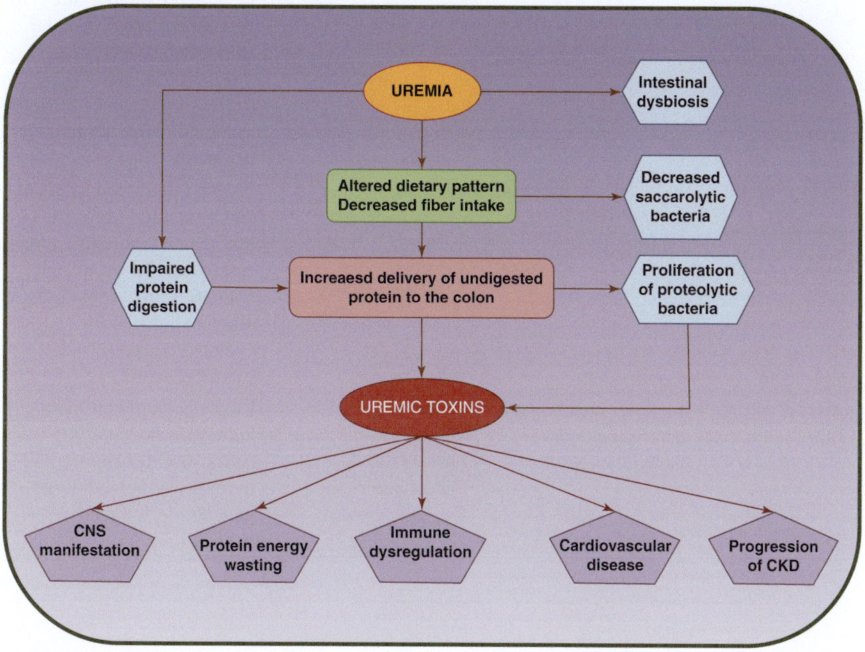

Fig. 4.1 Schematic representation of the association between uremia, dysbiotic gut microbiome, gut-derived uremic toxins, and the clinical manifestations of these uremic toxins [24]

Table 4.1 Metabolites associated with dysbiosis in chronic kidney disease [39–50]

Metabolites	Source	Associated bacteria	Remarks
Ammonia [42]	Bacterial hydrolysis of urea by urease; bacterial fermentation of glutamine, serine, threonine, and glycine	Urease is produced by several bacterial species including *Clostridioides* species, *Enterococcus*, *Shigella*, and *Escherichia coli*	High concentration of ammonia changes the luminal pH causing uremic colitis; amino acid catabolism leads to formation of sulfides, phenolic compounds, and amines, which are inflammatory and/or precursors to the formation of carcinogens
Hydrogen sulfide [43]	Reduction of sulfate and oxidized sulfur compounds, sulfur-containing amino acids such as cysteine	Sulfate-reducing bacteria *Escherichia coli*, *Salmonella enterica*, *Clostridioides*, and *Enterobacter aerogenes* convert cysteine to H_2S	Vasodilation, decreases inflammation, and renal fibrosis
Indoxyl sulfate [39]	Bacterial metabolism of tryptophan	*Clostridium sporogenes*, *E. coli*	Associated with increased vascular stiffness, aortic calcification, and cardiovascular mortality; increased oxidative stress in endothelial cells; vascular smooth muscle cell proliferation; and expression of genes related to tubulointerstitial fibrosis in kidney
Indole-3-acetic acid [41]	Endogenous; bacterial metabolism of tryptophan	*Clostridioides sporogenes*, *C. bartlettii*, *E. coli*	Induce glomerular sclerosis and interstitial fibrosis; predictor of mortality and cardiovascular events in patients with chronic kidney disease; induces cyclooxygenase-2 and oxidative stress
p-Cresyl sulfate [39]	Bacterial metabolism of tyrosine and phenylalanine	*Clostridioides difficile*, *F. prausnitzii*, *Bifidobacterium*, *Subdoligranulum*, *Lactobacillus*	Progression of chronic kidney disease, cardiovascular disease and mortality in hemodialysis patients; endothelial dysfunction

Table 4.1 (continued)

Metabolites	Source	Associated bacteria	Remarks
Phenylacetic acid [44]	Endogenous; bacterial metabolism of tryptophan	*Clostridioides* species, *Bacteroides* species	Toxic; induces nausea, vomiting, diarrhea and convulsion; associated with impaired immunoregulation, increased oxidative stress, and osteoblast dysfunction; causes renal tubular damage in dogs
1-Methyl guanidine [45]	Metabolism of creatinine	*Pseudomonas stutzeri*	Accumulate in chronic kidney disease. In rats with kidney failure dose-dependent increase in mortality
Trimethylamine N-oxide (TMAO) [46, 51]	Bacterial metabolism of dietary lipid phosphatidylcholine	*Faecalibacterium prausnitzii*, *Bifidobacterium*	Progression of kidney disease and mortality in chronic kidney disease. Associated with tubulointerstitial fibrosis, atherosclerotic vascular disease, heart failure, mortality in general population. Some evidence linking it to cardiovascular disease in chronic kidney disease patients
D-lactic acid [47]	Endogenous; bacterial production	*Enterococcus* and *Streptococcus* species	D-lactic acidosis; neurotoxic effects
Hippuric acid [48]	Ingestion, bacterial metabolism of aromatic compounds and polyphenols	*Clostridioides* species	Anion gap acidosis; may cause glucose intolerance and interfere with erythropoiesis and platelet cyclo-oxygenase activity
Short-chain fatty acid [49, 50]	Fermentation of complex polysaccharides	Most enteric bacteria, especially phyla Bacteroidetes and Firmicutes	Histone deacetylase inhibitors, regulate blood pressure and immune responses, protect against acute kidney injury

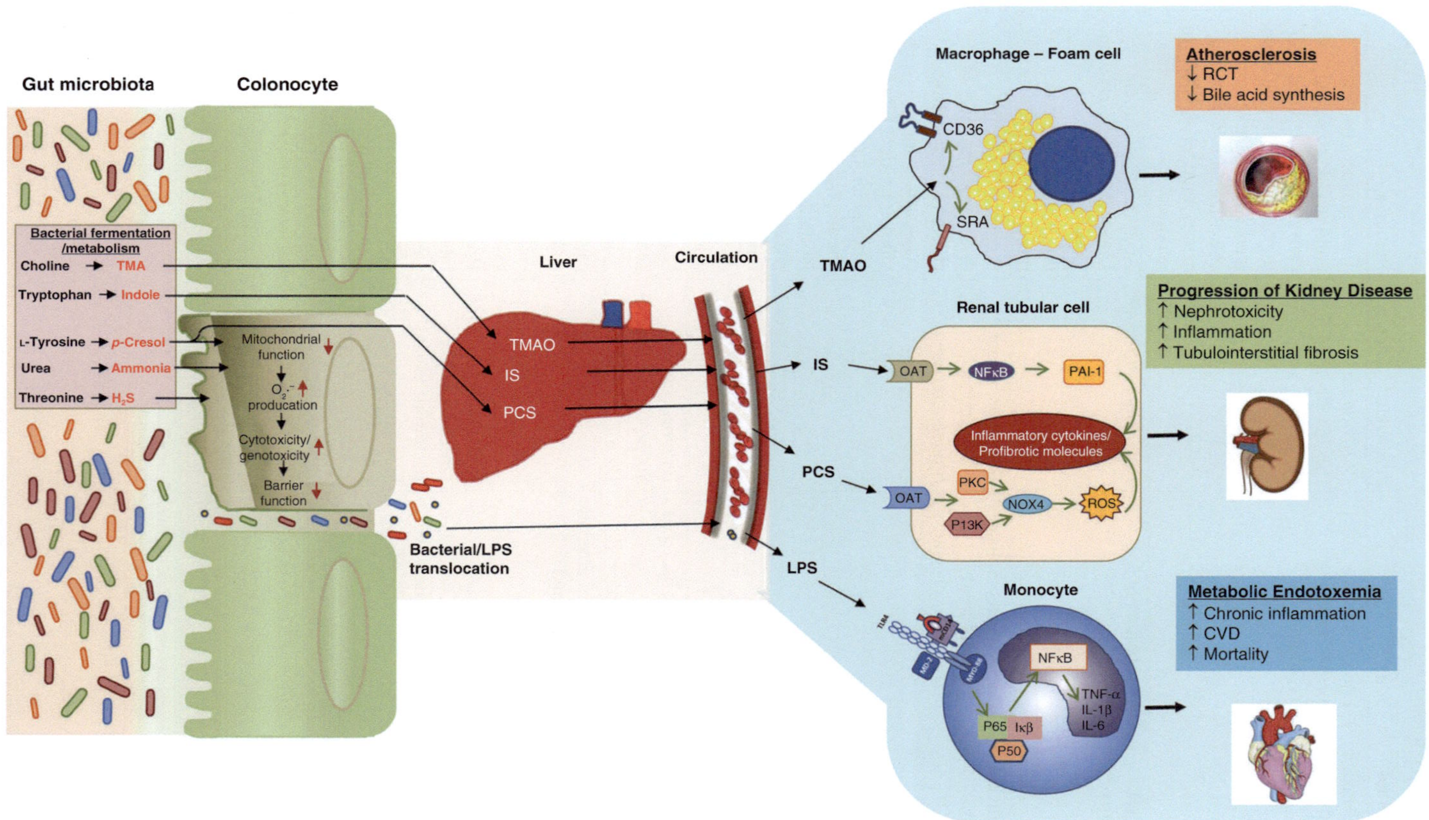

Fig. 4.2 Schematic representation of key toxic metabolites stemming from gut dysbiosis and their downstream pathways leading to pathophysiological consequences in chronic kidney disease [24]

Inflammation

Given its role in driving cardiovascular morbidity and CKD, mitigating systemic inflammation and oxidative stress is a desirable objective with the microbiome presenting opportune targets [52, 53]. Alterations in various pro-inflammatory and anti-inflammatory mediators have indeed been defined in dysbiotic states.

Richard Pfeiffer discovered a heat-stable toxin localized inside the bacterial cell and thus named it endotoxin to distinguish it from the already known exotoxins. Endotoxin is continuously produced in the gut and is transported into intestinal capillaries through a TLR4-dependent mechanism. Endotoxin provokes a host of responses by binding to the CD14 receptor [54, 55]. Elevation in the concentration of soluble CD14 (sCD14), an indicator of CD14 receptor activation, is an independent predictor of mortality among patients treated with maintenance hemodialysis [54, 55]. Endotoxin stimulates the immune system, particularly macrophages and the endothelial cells, to become activated and to synthesize and secrete a variety of effector molecules that cause an inflammatory response. Recent studies have detected microbial DNA in the blood of healthy individuals, a space traditionally considered microbe-free. Shah and colleagues showed that there is a qualitative differences in the circulating microbiome profile with significant taxonomic variations in the blood microbiome in patients with CKD compared with healthy controls [56].

The pro-inflammatory breakdown product p-cresol sulfate (metabolized by tryptophanase and hydroxyphenylacetate decarboxylase) is increased in advanced CKD due in part to over-abundance of phenol generating microbes and from reduced renal clearance itself [26, 57]. Such microbes include *Clostridium difficile*, *Lactobacillus*, and *Proteus vulgaris* [58–60].

Hydrogen sulfide, while not universally cytoprotective, does have important antioxidant properties in most physiologic states [61]. It has been shown to protect against renal fibrosis, and was also found to be lowered in an animal model of CKD thus underscoring its importance in this clinical setting [62, 63]. Moreover its role in modulating epithelial cell-mucus bacterial interactions and preventing gut dysbiosis has also been described [64]. Predominant sources involve degradation of sulfur-containing amino acids by colonic anaerobic bacteria such as *Escherichia coli*, *Salmonella enterica*, *Clostridia*, and *Enterobacter aerogenes* [65].

Immune Dysregulation

There have been numerous observations that demonstrate the gut microbiome's role in host adaptive and innate immunologic development. Central to this concept, is the dependence of naive T-cells on gut microbial antigen presentation in order to efficiently mature into Foxp3+ T-regulatory (Treg) cells [66]. Microbe generated SCFAs have been implicated in the regulation of T-cell differentiation into effector and Treg cells depending on their cytokinetic conditions [67]. Round and Mazmanian also defined polysaccharide A (produced by *Bacterioides fragilis*) as a key mediator in Treg maturation process in generating a more tolerogenic phenotype [68]. Atarshi and colleagues demonstrated similar properties of *Clostridia* in driving Treg cell development and hypothesized that metabolic intermediates were also at play [69]. Furthermore, the gut mucosal membrane's symbiotic relationship via metabolic pathways is exemplified by its dependence on *Bifidobacteria* and *Bacteroides* species to produce proprionate and butyrate which serve as nutrients for intestinal epithelial cells [70]. It is conceivable that gut dysbiosis may disrupt these intricate relationships, however, further work is needed to identify the precise microbial phenotype and its metabolites in CKD.

Hypertension

There is extensive animal and human data linking gut dysbiotic states with systemic arterial hypertension [71–74]. SCFAs such propionate and butyrate have exhibited vasorelaxant properties both in vitro and in human colonic arteries [75, 76]. Acetate has long been known for its vasodilatory actions, and is interestingly still attributed as the cause for intra-dialytic hypotension seen with acetate-buffered solutions [77–79]. There is also evidence that SCFAs mediate blood pressure changes via the juxtaglomerular apparatus through olfactory receptor 78 (Olfr78) and G protein-coupled receptor 41 (Gpr41) where they are known to be expressed [80]. This concept was consolidated in experiments using Olfr78 knockout mice that developed elevated blood pressure upon antibiotic-eradication of their gut microbiota [81]. High-salt diet has been shown to deplete *Lactobacillus murinus* and treatment of mice with *L. murinus* reduced T_H17 cell numbers and prevented salt-sensitive hypertension [82].

Progression of Kidney Disease

Efforts to understand mechanisms of CKD progression have led to the discovery of various pathways involving cytokines, transcription, and epigenetic factors as well metabolic mediators [83, 84]. Niwa and colleagues proposed the protein metabolite hypothesis, which claims that toxins generated from protein putrefaction by gut microbes are taken up by the organic anion transporters in the renal tubules, which activates cellular pathways leading to cell death and interstitial fibrosis [85].

A well studied mediator is indole, a product of tryptophan metabolism via tryptophanase expressing bacteria such as *E. coli*. Indole is metabolized into indoxyl sulfate (IS) through microsomal cytochrome P450 isozymes in the liver [86]. IS in turn may function as an aryl hydrocarbon receptor ligand and a transcriptional regulator [87]. Animal data suggests that IS may be associated with renal tubular and podocyte injury, as well as transcription factors driving tubulointerstitial fibrosis including TGF-β1 [88–90].

A second pathway towards progressive renal disease involves P-Cresol, a breakdown product of tyrosine and phenylalanine [87]. Using an animal model, Sun and colleagues showed that both IS and P-Cresol promoted renal fibrosis via several mechanisms including activation of the RAAS and TGF-β pathways along with inducing epithelial-to-mesenchymal transition by expression of the transcription factor, Snail [91]. The aforementioned experimental findings were substantiated in an observational study of some 268 CKD patients, in whom baseline IS and P-Cresol levels correlated with CKD progression [39].

Finally, Trimethylamine-*N*-oxide (TMAO) - a product of dietary choline, phosphatidylcholine (lecithin), and l-carnitine metabolism is also known to be elevated in CKD and has been linked with cardiovascular disease [92]. It is associated with diets rich in animal proteins and gut microbiota harboring *Prevotella* and *Acinetobacter* species [51, 93]. Tang and colleagues demonstrated its role in promoting renal fibrosis and dysfunction in mice fed with diets rich in choline [94]. The same group also reported poorer overall survival in individuals with elevated TMAO levels in CKD. Taken together, a causal link with TMAO levels and progressive renal disease is conceivable but remains to be proven.

Cardiovascular Disease

The interplay between gut dysbiosis and long-term cardiovascular risk is now well appreciated. Various microbiotic derivatives have been implicated in this process. An observational study of some 4007 coronary angiography candidates found elevations in levels of TMAO to be associated with incident major adverse cardiovascular events at 3 years of follow-up [40]. While this study was not limited to individuals with CKD, its applicability is supported in that higher TMAO levels are seen in this patient population. The tryptophan end-product, indole-3 acetic acid (IAA) was an independent predictor of cardiovascular events among CKD patients in an undertaking where the investigators ascribed it to its pro-oxidant and pro-inflammatory effects [41, 95]. Free p-cresol has also been associated with cardiovascular risk in both pre-dialysis and dialysis-dependent individuals [96, 97].

Obesity and Insulin Resistance

A widely accepted paradigm integrating intestinal inflammation with obesity and insulin resistance has drawn efforts to define microbiotic mediators of these endpoints [98]. This concept has been buoyed by experiments in which gut microbial transfers enriched with *Bacteroidetes* and the *Firmicutes* augmented dietary energy extraction resulting in obesity in a mouse model of dysbiosis [9]. Subsequent work from Ding and colleagues implicated inflammatory pathways including TNF-α and NF-κB in the development of obesity among conventional versus germ-free mice fed a high fat diet, supporting the role of both dysbiosis and inflammation in this process [99].

Molecular analysis has also revealed differing microbiotic profiles among diabetic and non-diabetic individuals. This includes lower representation in *B. vulgatus*, *Bifidobacterium*, *Firmicutes*, *Clostridia*, and universal butyrate-producing bacteria, along with enrichment in class *Betaproteobacteria* and certain opportunistic pathogens among diabetic subjects [100–102]. It has been hypothesized that dysbiosis-induced gut permeability coupled with systemic inflammation drives this insulin resistant phenotype [103–106]. This concept is supported through work by Cani and colleagues whereby increases in LPS was associated with obesity-associated insulin resistance and has been coined 'metabolic endotoxemia' [107–109].

Microbiome Therapeutics

The scientific community has sought to capitalize on the metabolic potential of microbiome through probiotics, prebiotics, xenobiotics, nutritional modifications, and genetically engineered bacteria with varying levels of success [110–113]. Prebiotics are microbial feed supplements that increase the intestinal growth of beneficial bacteria such as *Bifidobacteria*. Probiotics are living, non-pathogenic microorganisms that have beneficial health effects such as *Bifidobacteria* and *Lactobacilli*. Synbiotics are combinations of prebiotics and probiotics (refer to Table 4.2). In PD

Table 4.2 Effect of probiotic, prebiotic, and synbiotic therapy in kidney disease [27, 48, 114–122]

Reference	Patient (*n*)	Intervention	Response
Nakabayashi [114]	HD (7)	Galacto-oligosaccharides + *L. casei*, and *B. breve*	↓ PCS
Pavan [115]	CKD (24)	Probiotic and prebiotic	↓ CKD progression
Guida [116]	CKD (30)	Probiotic + inulin and resistant starch	↓ PCS
Rossi [117]	CKD (37)	Probiotic + prebiotic (inulin and galactooligosaccarides)	↓ PCS
Meijers [118]	HD (22)	Oligofructose-enriched inulin	↓ PCS
Cruz-Mora [119]	HD (18)	*L. acidophilus* and *B. lactis* + inulin	↑ Bifidobacteria
Viramontes-Hörner [120]	HD (42)	*L. aidophilus* and *B. lactis* + inulin	↓ CRP (trend)
Wang [121]	PD (39)	*B. bifidum*, *B. catenulatum*, *B. longum*, and *L. plantarum*	↓TNF-α, IL-6, LPS
Takayama [122]	HD (22)	*Bifidobacterium longum*	↓ IS
Hida [27]	HD (25)	*Bifidobacterium infantis*, *Lactobacillus acidophilus*, *Enterococcus faecalis*	↓ p-Cresol in feces
Andrade-Oliveira [48]	Mice	*B. adolescentis* or *B. longum*	↑ Acetate; Protects mice from AKI

patients, treatment with prebiotic, oligofructose-enriched p-inulin altered microbial co-metabolism, with significant reduction in TMAO concentration [28]. Unfortunately, there are no well-designed large scale studies examining the role of microbiome-based therapy in kidney disease to draw any meaningful conclusions.

Bioengineering approaches can be used for reshaping the dysbiotic microbiome and engineered smart microbes could be used to detect and treat disease [123]. In an elegant study, Delvin and colleagues showed that indoxyl sulfate levels could be reduced by changing the abundance or the microbial enzyme (tryptophanases) involved in generation of the metabolites [57].

Conclusion

Rapid advances in DNA sequencing technology resulted have accelerated identification of the community structure and functional capability of microbiome in human health and disease. Dysbiotic states have been causally linked to several metabolic and inflammatory diseases, including atherosclerosis. Unfortunately, the lack of large scale metagenomic data has greatly impeded progress in our understanding of microbiome in kidney disease. In health, the gut microbiome exists in "symbiosis," a state of coexistence in mutual harmony. This metabolic synergy is disturbed in CKD, leading to generation of uremic toxins and excess inflammation. In 2018 alone, over 2400 clinical trials were testing therapies based on microbiome science and nephrology is lagging in well-designed and adequately powered studies. With evidence mounting of the gut microbiome's health significance, synthetic biologists are looking to engineer the microbiome. The quest for microbiome-based therapy for CKD continues with some very preliminary hint of hope.

References

1. Tabrett A, Horton MW. The influence of host genetics on the microbiome. F1000Res. 2020;9:84.
2. David LA, et al. Diet rapidly and reproducibly alters the human gut microbiome. Nature. 2014;505(7484):559–63.
3. Maier L, et al. Extensive impact of non-antibiotic drugs on human gut bacteria. Nature. 2018;555(7698):623–8.
4. Rothschild D, et al. Environment dominates over host genetics in shaping human gut microbiota. Nature. 2018;555(7695):210–5.
5. Huttenhower C, et al. Structure, function and diversity of the healthy human microbiome. Nature. 2012;486(7402):207–14.
6. Turnbaugh PJ, et al. The human microbiome project. Nature. 2007;449(7164):804–10.
7. Qin J, et al. A human gut microbial gene catalogue established by metagenomic sequencing. Nature. 2010;464(7285):59–65.
8. Eloe-Fadrosh EA, Rasko DA. The human microbiome: from symbiosis to pathogenesis. Annu Rev Med. 2013;64:145–63.

9. Turnbaugh PJ, et al. An obesity-associated gut microbiome with increased capacity for energy harvest. Nature. 2006;444(7122):1027–31.
10. Krajmalnik-Brown R, et al. Effects of gut microbes on nutrient absorption and energy regulation. Nutr Clin Pract. 2012;27(2):201–14.
11. Vrieze A, et al. Transfer of intestinal microbiota from lean donors increases insulin sensitivity in individuals with metabolic syndrome. Gastroenterology. 2012;143(4):913–6.
12. Belkaid Y, Hand TW. Role of the microbiota in immunity and inflammation. Cell. 2014;157(1):121–41.
13. Kriss M, et al. Low diversity gut microbiota dysbiosis: drivers, functional implications and recovery. Curr Opin Microbiol. 2018;44:34–40.
14. Magnusson M, et al. Increased intestinal permeability to differently sized polyethylene glycols in uremic rats: effects of low- and high-protein diets. Nephron. 1990;56(3):306–11.
15. Magnusson M, et al. Impaired intestinal barrier function measured by differently sized polyethylene glycols in patients with chronic renal failure. Gut. 1991;32(7):754–9.
16. Ley RE, et al. Microbial ecology: human gut microbes associated with obesity. Nature. 2006;444(7122):1022–3.
17. Musso G, Gambino R, Cassader M. Interactions between gut microbiota and host metabolism predisposing to obesity and diabetes. Annu Rev Med. 2011;62(1):361–80.
18. Sun M, et al. Regulatory immune cells in regulation of intestinal inflammatory response to microbiota. Mucosal Immunol. 2015;8(5):969–78.
19. Sampson TR, et al. Gut microbiota regulate motor deficits and neuroinflammation in a model of Parkinson's disease. Cell. 2016;167(6):1469–80.
20. Singh V, et al. Microbiota dysbiosis controls the neuroinflammatory response after stroke. J Neurosci. 2016;36(28):7428–40.
21. Berer K, et al. Gut microbiota from multiple sclerosis patients enables spontaneous autoimmune encephalomyelitis in mice. Proc Natl Acad Sci. 2017;114(40):10719.
22. Carlson AL, et al. Infant gut microbiome associated with cognitive development. Biol Psychiatry. 2018;83(2):148–59.
23. Li Y, et al. Dysbiosis of the gut microbiome is associated with CKD5 and correlated with clinical indices of the disease: a case–controlled study. J Transl Med. 2019;17(1):228.
24. Ramezani A, et al. Role of the gut microbiome in uremia: a potential therapeutic target. Am J Kidney Dis. 2016;67(3):483–98.
25. Vaziri ND, et al. Chronic kidney disease alters intestinal microbial flora. Kidney Int. 2013;83(2):308–15.
26. Wong J, et al. Expansion of urease- and uricase-containing, indole- and p-cresol-forming and contraction of short-chain fatty acid-producing intestinal microbiota in ESRD. Am J Nephrol. 2014;39(3):230–7.
27. Hida M, et al. Inhibition of the accumulation of uremic toxins in the blood and their precursors in the feces after oral administration of Lebenin, a lactic acid bacteria preparation, to uremic patients undergoing hemodialysis. Nephron. 1996;74(2):349–55.
28. Gao B, et al. A pilot study on the effect of prebiotic on host-microbial co-metabolism in peritoneal dialysis patients. Kidney Int Rep. 2020;5(8):1309–15.
29. Rohan P, Dominic SR. Metabolic synergy to uremic toxicity: a tale of symbiosis and dysbiosis in CKD. Nephrology. 2019;18(4):187–93.
30. Kang JY. The gastrointestinal tract in uremia. Dig Dis Sci. 1993;38(2):257–68.
31. Kalantar-Zadeh K, et al. Food intake characteristics of hemodialysis patients as obtained by food frequency questionnaire. J Ren Nutr. 2002;12(1):17–31.
32. Jernberg C, et al. Long-term impacts of antibiotic exposure on the human intestinal microbiota. Microbiology. 2010;156(11):3216–23.
33. Wu MJ, et al. Colonic transit time in long-term dialysis patients. Am J Kidney Dis. 2004;44(2):322–7.
34. Gao B, Regunathan R, Shrivastava A, Barrows IR, Amdur RL, Andrews SC, Raj DS. Gut microbiota and host co-metabolism are altered by patiromer induced changes in serum and stool potassium. Kidney Int Rep. 2021;6(3):821–9.

35. Farhadi A, et al. Intestinal barrier: an interface between health and disease. J Gastroenterol Hepatol. 2003;18(5):479–97.
36. de Almeida Duarte JB, et al. Bacterial translocation in experimental uremia. Urol Res. 2004;32(4):266–70.
37. Cummings JH, et al. The effect of meat protein and dietary fiber on colonic function and metabolism. II. Bacterial metabolites in feces and urine. Am J Clin Nutr. 1979;32(10):2094–101.
38. Smith EA, Macfarlane GT. Studies on amine production in the human colon: enumeration of amine forming bacteria and physiological effects of carbohydrate and pH. Anaerobe. 1996;2(5):285–97.
39. Wu IW, et al. p-Cresyl sulphate and indoxyl sulphate predict progression of chronic kidney disease. Nephrol Dial Transplant. 2011;26(3):938–47.
40. Tang WH, et al. Intestinal microbial metabolism of phosphatidylcholine and cardiovascular risk. N Engl J Med. 2013;368(17):1575–84.
41. Dou L, et al. The cardiovascular effect of the uremic solute indole-3 acetic acid. J Am Soc Nephrol. 2015;26(4):876–87.
42. Kingsbury FB, Swanson WW. The synthesis and elimination of hippuric acid in nephritis: a new renal function test: preliminary paper. Arch Intern Med. 1921;28(2):220–36.
43. Macfarlane GT, Cummings JH, Allison C. Protein degradation by human intestinal bacteria. J Gen Microbiol. 1986;132(6):1647–56.
44. Brooks DP, et al. Production of methylguanidine in dogs with acute and chronic renal failure. Clin Sci. 1989;77(6):637–41.
45. Jankowski J, et al. Increased plasma phenylacetic acid in patients with end-stage renal failure inhibits iNOS expression. J Clin Invest. 2003;112(2):256–64.
46. Perna A, Ingrosso D. Low hydrogen sulphide and chronic kidney disease: a dangerous liaison. Nephrol Dial Transplant. 2012;27:486–93.
47. Arpaia N, et al. Metabolites produced by commensal bacteria promote peripheral regulatory T-cell generation. Nature. 2013;504(7480):451–5.
48. Andrade-Oliveira V, et al. Gut bacteria products prevent AKI induced by ischemia-reperfusion. J Am Soc Nephrol. 2015;26(8):1877–88.
49. Stubbs JR, et al. Serum trimethylamine-N-oxide is elevated in CKD and correlates with coronary atherosclerosis burden. J Am Soc Nephrol. 2016;27(1):305–13.
50. Yilmaz B, et al. D-lactic acidosis: successful suppression of D-lactate-producing Lactobacillus by probiotics. Pediatrics. 2018;142:3.
51. Wang Z, et al. Gut flora metabolism of phosphatidylcholine promotes cardiovascular disease. Nature. 2011;472(7341):57–63.
52. Stenvinkel P, et al. Strong association between malnutrition, inflammation, and atherosclerosis in chronic renal failure. Kidney Int. 1999;55(5):1899–911.
53. Amdur RL, et al. Inflammation and progression of CKD: the CRIC study. Clin J Am Soc Nephrol. 2016;11(9):1546–56.
54. Raj DS, et al. Soluble CD14 levels, interleukin 6, and mortality among prevalent hemodialysis patients. Am J Kidney Dis. 2009;54(6):1072–80.
55. Raj DS, et al. Association of soluble endotoxin receptor CD14 and mortality among patients undergoing hemodialysis. Am J Kidney Dis. 2009;54(6):1062–71.
56. Mair RD, Sirich TL. Blood microbiome in CKD: should we care? Clin J Am Soc Nephrol. 2019;14(5):648–9.
57. Devlin AS, et al. Modulation of a circulating uremic solute via rational genetic manipulation of the gut microbiota. Cell Host Microbe. 2016;20(6):709–15.
58. Yokoyama MT, Carlson JR. Production of skatole and para-cresol by a rumen Lactobacillus sp. Appl Environ Microbiol. 1981;41(1):71–6.
59. Ward LA, et al. Isolation from swine feces of a bacterium which decarboxylates p-hydroxyphenylacetic acid to 4-methylphenol (p-cresol). Appl Environ Microbiol. 1987;53(1):189–92.

60. Selmer T, Andrei PI. p-Hydroxyphenylacetate decarboxylase from Clostridium difficile. A novel glycyl radical enzyme catalysing the formation of p-cresol. Eur J Biochem. 2001;268(5):1363–72.
61. Predmore BL, Lefer DJ, Gojon G. Hydrogen sulfide in biochemistry and medicine. Antioxid Redox Signal. 2012;17(1):119–40.
62. Aminzadeh MA, Vaziri ND. Downregulation of the renal and hepatic hydrogen sulfide (H2S)-producing enzymes and capacity in chronic kidney disease. Nephrol Dial Transplant. 2012;27(2):498–504.
63. Song K, et al. Hydrogen sulfide inhibits the renal fibrosis of obstructive nephropathy. Kidney Int. 2014;85(6):1318–29.
64. Wallace JL, Motta JP, Buret AG. Hydrogen sulfide: an agent of stability at the microbiome-mucosa interface. Am J Physiol Gastrointest Liver Physiol. 2018;314(2):143–9.
65. Blachier F, et al. Luminal sulfide and large intestine mucosa: friend or foe? Amino Acids. 2010;39(2):335–47.
66. Lathrop SK, et al. Peripheral education of the immune system by colonic commensal microbiota. Nature. 2011;478(7368):250–4.
67. Park J, et al. Short-chain fatty acids induce both effector and regulatory T cells by suppression of histone deacetylases and regulation of the mTOR-S6K pathway. Mucosal Immunol. 2015;8(1):80–93.
68. Round JL, Mazmanian SK. Inducible Foxp3+ regulatory T-cell development by a commensal bacterium of the intestinal microbiota. Proc Natl Acad Sci U S A. 2010;107(27):12204–9.
69. Atarashi K, et al. Induction of colonic regulatory T cells by indigenous Clostridium species. Science. 2011;331(6015):337–41.
70. Maynard CL, et al. Reciprocal interactions of the intestinal microbiota and immune system. Nature. 2012;489(7415):231–41.
71. Jose PA, Raj D. Gut microbiota in hypertension. Curr Opin Nephrol Hypertens. 2015;24(5):403–9.
72. Mell B, et al. Evidence for a link between gut microbiota and hypertension in the Dahl rat. Physiol Genomics. 2015;47(6):187–97.
73. Yang T, et al. Gut dysbiosis is linked to hypertension. Hypertension. 2015;65(6):1331–40.
74. Durgan DJ, et al. Role of the gut microbiome in obstructive sleep apnea-induced hypertension. Hypertension. 2016;67(2):469–74.
75. Mortensen FV, et al. Short chain fatty acids dilate isolated human colonic resistance arteries. Gut. 1990;31(12):1391–4.
76. Pevsner-Fischer M, et al. The gut microbiome and hypertension. Curr Opin Nephrol Hypertens. 2017;26(1):1–8.
77. Bauer W, Richards DW. A vasodilator action of acetates. J Physiol. 1928;66(4):371–8.
78. Keshaviah PR. The role of acetate in the etiology of symptomatic hypotension. Artif Organs. 1982;6(4):378–87.
79. Saragoca MA, et al. Sodium acetate, an arterial vasodilator: haemodynamic characterisation in normal dogs. Proc Eur Dial Transplant Assoc Eur Ren Assoc. 1985;21:221–4.
80. Pluznick JL, et al. Functional expression of the olfactory signaling system in the kidney. Proc Natl Acad Sci. 2009;106(6):2059.
81. Pluznick JL, et al. Olfactory receptor responding to gut microbiota-derived signals plays a role in renin secretion and blood pressure regulation. Proc Natl Acad Sci. 2013;110(11):4410.
82. Wilck N, et al. Salt-responsive gut commensal modulates T(H)17 axis and disease. Nature. 2017;551(7682):585–9.
83. Rhee EP, et al. Metabolomics of chronic kidney disease progression: a case-control analysis in the chronic renal insufficiency cohort study. Am J Nephrol. 2016;43(5):366–74.
84. Ruiz-Ortega M, et al. Targeting the progression of chronic kidney disease. Nat Rev Nephrol. 2020;16(5):269–88.
85. Niwa T. Organic acids and the uremic syndrome: protein metabolite hypothesis in the progression of chronic renal failure. Semin Nephrol. 1996;16(3):167–82.

86. Banoglu E, Jha GG, King RS. Hepatic microsomal metabolism of indole to indoxyl, a precursor of indoxyl sulfate. Eur J Drug Metab Pharmacokinet. 2001;26(4):235–40.
87. Nallu A, et al. Gut microbiome in chronic kidney disease: challenges and opportunities. Transl Res. 2017;179:24–37.
88. Miyazaki T, et al. Indoxyl sulfate increases the gene expressions of TGF-beta 1, TIMP-1 and pro-alpha 1(I) collagen in uremic rat kidneys. Kidney Int Suppl. 1997;62:15–22.
89. Satoh M, et al. Uremic toxins overload accelerates renal damage in a rat model of chronic renal failure. Nephron Exp Nephrol. 2003;95(3):e111–8.
90. Ichii O, et al. Podocyte injury caused by indoxyl sulfate, a uremic toxin and aryl-hydrocarbon receptor ligand. PLoS One. 2014;9(9):e108448.
91. Sun CY, Chang SC, Wu MS. Uremic toxins induce kidney fibrosis by activating intrarenal renin-angiotensin-aldosterone system associated epithelial-to-mesenchymal transition. PLoS One. 2012;7(3):e34026.
92. Moraes C, et al. Trimethylamine N-oxide from gut microbiota in chronic kidney disease patients: focus on diet. J Ren Nutr. 2015;25(6):459–65.
93. Koeth RA, et al. Intestinal microbiota metabolism of l-carnitine, a nutrient in red meat, promotes atherosclerosis. Nat Med. 2013;19(5):576–85.
94. Tang WH, et al. Gut microbiota-dependent trimethylamine N-oxide (TMAO) pathway contributes to both development of renal insufficiency and mortality risk in chronic kidney disease. Circ Res. 2015;116(3):448–55.
95. Jourde-Chiche N, et al. Protein-bound toxins–update. Semin Dial. 2009;22(4):334–9.
96. Meijers BK, et al. Free p-cresol is associated with cardiovascular disease in hemodialysis patients. Kidney Int. 2008;73(10):1174–80.
97. Meijers BK, et al. p-Cresol and cardiovascular risk in mild-to-moderate kidney disease. Clin J Am Soc Nephrol. 2010;5(7):1182–9.
98. Ding S, Lund PK. Role of intestinal inflammation as an early event in obesity and insulin resistance. Curr Opin Clin Nutr Metab Care. 2011;14(4):328–33.
99. Ding S, et al. High-fat diet: bacteria interactions promote intestinal inflammation which precedes and correlates with obesity and insulin resistance in mouse. PLoS One. 2010;5(8):e12191.
100. Larsen N, et al. Gut microbiota in human adults with type 2 diabetes differs from non-diabetic adults. PLoS One. 2010;5(2):e9085.
101. Wu X, et al. Molecular characterisation of the faecal microbiota in patients with type II diabetes. Curr Microbiol. 2010;61(1):69–78.
102. Qin J, et al. A metagenome-wide association study of gut microbiota in type 2 diabetes. Nature. 2012;490(7418):55–60.
103. Diamant M, Blaak EE, de Vos WM. Do nutrient-gut-microbiota interactions play a role in human obesity, insulin resistance and type 2 diabetes? Obes Rev. 2011;12(4):272–81.
104. Everard A, Cani PD. Diabetes, obesity and gut microbiota. Best Pract Res Clin Gastroenterol. 2013;27(1):73–83.
105. Lee J. Adipose tissue macrophages in the development of obesity-induced inflammation, insulin resistance and type 2 diabetes. Arch Pharm Res. 2013;36(2):208–22.
106. McArdle MA, et al. Mechanisms of obesity-induced inflammation and insulin resistance: insights into the emerging role of nutritional strategies. Front Endocrinol. 2013;4:52.
107. Cani PD, et al. Metabolic endotoxemia initiates obesity and insulin resistance. Diabetes. 2007;56(7):1761.
108. Cani PD, et al. Changes in gut microbiota control metabolic endotoxemia-induced inflammation in high-fat diet-induced obesity and diabetes in mice. Diabetes. 2008;57(6):1470–81.
109. Cani PD, et al. Role of gut microflora in the development of obesity and insulin resistance following high-fat diet feeding. Pathol Biol. 2008;56(5):305–9.
110. Jain P, et al. Potentials and limitations of microorganisms as renal failure biotherapeutics. Biol Theory. 2009;3:233–43.

111. Cosola C, et al. Nutrients, nutraceuticals, and xenobiotics affecting renal health. Nutrients. 2018;10(7):808.
112. Jia L, et al. Efficacy of probiotics supplementation on chronic kidney disease: a systematic review and meta-analysis. Kidney Blood Press Res. 2018;43(5):1623–35.
113. Bres E, Koppe L. Is there still a place for prebiotics in chronic kidney disease? Nephrol Dial Transplant. 2019;34(11):1812–6.
114. Takayama F, Taki K, Niwa T. Bifidobacterium in gastro-resistant seamless capsule reduces serum levels of indoxyl sulfate in patients on hemodialysis. Am J Kidney Dis. 2003;41(3):142–5.
115. Meijers BK, et al. p-Cresyl sulfate serum concentrations in haemodialysis patients are reduced by the prebiotic oligofructose-enriched inulin. Nephrol Dial Transplant. 2010;25(1):219–24.
116. Nakabayashi I, et al. Effects of synbiotic treatment on serum level of p-cresol in haemodialysis patients: a preliminary study. Nephrol Dial Transplant. 2011;26(3):1094–8.
117. Cruz-Mora J, et al. Effects of a symbiotic on gut microbiota in Mexican patients with end-stage renal disease. J Ren Nutr. 2014;24(5):330–5.
118. Guida B, et al. Effect of short-term synbiotic treatment on plasma p-cresol levels in patients with chronic renal failure: a randomized clinical trial. Nutr Metab Cardiovasc Dis. 2014;24(9):1043–9.
119. Rossi M, et al. SYNbiotics easing renal failure by improving Gut microbiologY (SYNERGY): a protocol of placebo-controlled randomised cross-over trial. BMC Nephrol. 2014;15:106.
120. Viramontes-Hörner D, et al. Effect of a symbiotic gel (Lactobacillus acidophilus + Bifidobacterium lactis + inulin) on presence and severity of gastrointestinal symptoms in hemodialysis patients. J Ren Nutr. 2015;25(3):284–91.
121. Wang IK, et al. The effect of probiotics on serum levels of cytokine and endotoxin in peritoneal dialysis patients: a randomised, double-blind, placebo-controlled trial. Benefic Microbes. 2015;6(4):423–30.
122. Pavan M. Influence of prebiotic and probiotic supplementation on the progression of chronic kidney disease. Minerva Urol Nefrol. 2016;68(2):222–6.
123. Sonnenburg JL. Microbiome engineering. Nature. 2015;518(7540):10.

Chapter 5
Psychological Factors Associated with Adjustment to Kidney Disease and Engagement in Novel Technologies

Stephanie Donahue, Eshika Kalam, and Daniel Cukor

Since the pioneering work of Selye [1] in describing the human stress response, the study of how people emotionally respond to challenge has flourished. McEwen and colleagues defined allostasis as the body's dynamic effort toward maintaining stability despite constant change [2]. Different types of stressors elicit different patterns of activation of the sympathetic nervous system, hypothalamic-pituitary-adrenocortical axis, and modulate negative feedback loops [3]. Understanding the person who is being impacted by kidney disease will help predict how that patient will respond to the physical and mental challenges as well as what types of interventions they will be likely to engage in, including their openness to the incorporation of novel technologies, a key personality construct in the ever-changing medical care environment.

Stress of Kidney Disease

Stress often accompanies chronic illness and its treatment, and may critically influence psychological and medical outcomes [4]. Chronic kidney disease (CKD) can be a stressful diagnosis with psychological challenges that include responding to intermittent acute stress on top of chronic illness, reduction in quality of life, demanding treatments that are lifelong and feelings of sadness, anxiety, and guilt. As a result, patients may present with stress related comorbid illnesses such as mood disorders, addiction disorders, chronic pain, sleep disturbances, as well as noncompliance to the medical prescriptions, decreased quality of life and increased morbidity and mortality [5].

S. Donahue · E. Kalam · D. Cukor (✉)
The Rogosin Institute, Behavioral Health, New York, NY, USA
e-mail: sld9001@nyp.org; esk9018@nyp.org; Dac9227@nyp.org

S. J. Saggi, M. O. Salifu (eds.), *Technological Advances in Care of Patients with Kidney Diseases*, https://doi.org/10.1007/978-3-031-11942-2_5

Symptom Burden

Studies have identified common symptoms reported in patients with CKD. Many patient symptom inventories describe the high burden in patients with ESRD [6, 7]. Harwood et al. found fatigue, sleep problems, peripheral neuropathy, muscle cramps, and restless legs to be the most commonly reported physical symptoms in patients with CKD [8]. They found the most frequently used and most effective coping strategy to be optimism. Confrontive (tackling a stressor head-on) and supportive (gaining support from others) coping styles were also used frequently and effectively [8]. In a recent national survey of patients with ESRD being treated with dialysis, patients identified fatigue, muscle cramps, and body aches as the most troublesome physical symptoms and depression, frustration, and anxiety as the most troublesome emotional symptoms [9].

Treatment Demands of CKD/ESRD

Beyond the toll that ESRD can take on the patient's body and mind, treatment itself can be quite onerous. Treatment demands in patients with CKD can cause side effects, alter daily life and cause stress for the patient and their caregiver. They generally include treatment for the sequelae of chronic kidney disease including oral medications, injections, infusions, diet restrictions and sometimes surgery for issues like hypertension, anemia, mineral imbalance, secondary hyperparathyroidism, fluid overload, and renal failure. Patients are also required to attend frequent medical appointments which is both time consuming and costly in many cases. All of this, with the constant awareness that kidney failure would necessitate renal replacement therapy.

Etiology of Depression and Anxiety in CKD and ESRD

The high symptom and treatment burden for patients with CKD can take an emotional toll and place them at risk for the development of psychopathology. Patients who are constantly fatigued, feeling ill, and have a high demand illness are at a greater risk for developing depression and anxiety. The patient's coping style may also contribute to the onset or delay of depressed mood [10]. When patients feel that they have the emotional resources to handle the presented challenge they tend to respond with an optimistic, energized attitude. However, if people believe that the stressor's demands are greater than their resources to cope with them, depression and anxiety may ensue. Cognitive Behavioral Therapy (CBT) postulates that depression occurs when people have negativistic beliefs about themselves, and when these beliefs are consistent over time and have a broad scope [11]. For the patient with

ESRD, their condition is likely irreversible and quite demanding, which engenders beliefs that are likely to be negativistic, consistent, and broad in nature [12]. The key variable, then, appears to be in how the individual interprets the locus of their challenge. People who equate themselves with their illness would be at more risk for developing depression than those who can create some emotional distance between their "true self" and their illness [13]. The theory of learned helplessness has also been used to conceptualize the development of depression [14]. In this understanding, people who believe that no matter what they do, the outcome is immutable, they learn to not try and emotionally give up. As this model would be applied to patients with ESRD, the belief that poor health is inevitable despite all of the effort that a patient may put in, would serve as a cause for helplessness, hopelessness, and depression.

Epidemiology of Depression and Anxiety in CKD and ESRD

Depression and anxiety are common in patients with chronic kidney disease. Some estimates are above 80% for depression [15] and above 50% for anxiety [7]. This surpasses the estimates reported for the general population of a lifelong incidence of 20.6% for depression and 33.7% overall for anxiety [16]. Zalai et al. report "Mood disorders can be regarded as the final common pathway developing from the interaction among multiple pathophysiological, psychological, and socioeconomic stressors that chronic illness imposes on the individual." [17]. The potential impact of anxiety in patients with ESRD was reported by Schouten et al. who followed 687 hemodialysis patients. They found an increased risk of anxiety symptoms in these patients which was associated with all-cause mortality, and increased 1-year hospitalization rates and length of hospital stay [18]. These findings highlight that anxiety can be as significant a comorbidity as medical conditions in hemodialysis populations [19]. Additional outcomes of anxiety were examined by Feroze et al., who conducted a cross-sectional study and brief literature review assessing anxiety and depression in dialysis patients. They also noted a high prevalence of anxiety and depression in the patients studied, and found that health concerns, dialysis treatment and even the dialysis center can serve as triggers for anxiety [20]. Brito et al. [21] found that anxiety correlated with loss of vascular access in patients treated with hemodialysis [21]. In a study by Cukor et al. [22], an anxiety diagnosis was found in 45.7% of 70 patients treated with hemodialysis (HD) utilizing a standardized psychiatric interview. Hedayati et al. used the Veterans Administration database to identify 1588 male HD patients. The physician-diagnosed rate of depression was 14.7%. Over the course of 2 years, a diagnosis of depression was associated with more hospitalizations and increased duration of hospitalization [23]. Mapes et al. looked at data from 142 facilities in the United States and 101 facilities in Europe, with a sample size of 5256 patients and found that patients with depression had a 27% higher adjusted mortality risk and a 14% higher relative risk of hospitalization [24].

Mood disorders in patients with CKD are associated with decreased health related quality of life (HRQOL), and increased comorbid illness, hospitalization and mortality. HRQOL is a validated system of measuring patients' physical, mental, and social well-being. It is a significant variable in the evaluation of the patient with CKD and is shown to correlate with adverse events such as hospitalization and death. In the Dialysis Outcomes and Practice Patterns Study (DOPPS) Mapes et al. found that depressive symptoms and diagnoses of depression which reduced HRQOL, were found to be independently associated with increased risks of hospitalization and mortality. Mapes et al. suggest that "DOPPS data suggest that even a single question related to depression can help identify dialysis patients at higher risk of these adverse outcomes." [24]. As clinicians and payers focus more on a patient-centered care model, the evaluation and recognition of the importance of HRQOL is an important first step in the identification of factors which influence HRQOL as critical to survival.

The treatments for CKD and ESRD are complex, involved and often demanding. Patients with a willingness to engage in complex self-care behaviors and have an openness to novel technologies will continue to receive state-of-the-art care [25]. Just as psychological and emotional variables explain how a person will respond to the demands of their illness, similarly, cognitive and emotional factors can be used to understand the likelihood of a person accepting new medical technologies.

Health information technology has been identified as a key to improving population health outcomes and health care quality [26]. Technologies such as smart phones, laptops, and other transportable devices are constantly being used to provide information and educational support programs for patients. Patient education is well known to improve outcomes in patients with CKD but the National Health and Nutrition Examination Survey data suggests that overall awareness of CKD status among people with CKD was only 6.4% [27]. Technology is a way to reach a wide range of people on a broad range of topics and increase their awareness and understanding of CKD. Being able to use technology on a daily basis will allow patients to see the available information and promote patient independence and self-empowerment. Patients who are able to accept and utilize new technology will have better self-management, which can essentially improve quality of life and overall mental health for the patient. This is particularly important for patients with chronic illness such as chronic kidney disease. Furthermore, new technologies are assisting in early identification of kidney disease and monitoring its progression. This can be beneficial to physicians and patients as it allows patients to gain control over their chronic illness therefore increasing adherence and positive outcomes.

Technology Acceptance

Technology acceptance is a construct that is designed to measure how users begin to accept and use new technology. The technology acceptance model was designed to help understand, predict and ultimately increase technology acceptability among its users [28]. The model suggests that users are influenced by multiple cognitive factors when making a decision about adopting a new technology. The theory states that successful adoption of new technology depends upon the positive determination of two main factors: perceived usefulness and perceived ease of use. Perceived usefulness is defined as when one believes that utilizing the particular system will improve his/her performance. Perceived ease of use is when one believes that using the system will be effortless [28]. In addition to these factors, there are a variety of other factors that influence utilization and adoption of new technology, such as; age, gender, race, education, socioeconomic status, and access to technology. Technology use tends to be higher for those who are younger and with higher levels of education. Computer and internet use are much lower among the elderly, minorities, disabled people and people with lower socioeconomic status partly due to lack of access and familiarity. Elderly populations in particular report a lack of confidence in learning and utilizing new systems effectively, hence this population experiences a high level of computer anxiety. Furthermore, those with positive attitudes toward technology use, higher interest and higher level of self-efficacy are more likely to engage in technology use [29].

Technology Acceptance in Healthcare Settings

In healthcare settings, trust and privacy are additional factors that are important in determining a patient's intention of utilizing novel technology. Enhanced trust in the technology is directly associated with the patients' intention of incorporating it into their healthcare [30]. As with all technology, the perceived ease of use and the perceived utility of the new technology are key components in driving uptake. Privacy concerns introduce an additional component of perceived harm and will reduce patients' likelihood of engaging in novel technologies.

Technology Acceptance in CKD

There has been relatively little research examining the acceptance of technology in patients with CKD. Perhaps the most significant work to date on mobile technology acceptance in CKD has been done by Hussein et al. [31] who administered a survey based on the Khatun mobile health readiness conceptual model, to 949 dialysis patients, 632 in-center patients, and 317 home dialysis patients. The Khatun model assesses the availability of devices and the internet and the proficiency and interest in using mobile health. They found that 81% owned internet capable devices, 72% reported using the internet, and 70% reported intermediate or advanced mobile health proficiency. Their conclusion was that the majority of patients on dialysis were ready for and proficient in mobile health.

One of the areas that has received some attention is medication safety. Medication regimens that include multiple drugs can be difficult to follow especially in the setting of CKD. This can be especially true when the patient also experiences emotional and cognitive fluctuations associated with uremia. Laville et al. studied 3033 outpatients with CKD and found adverse drug reactions or ADRs reported at a rate of 14.4 per 100 person-years overall and 2.7 per 100 person-years for serious ADRs including death [32]. In an attempt to address medication errors, Ong et al. studied 182 outpatients with CKD and the effectiveness of two digital applications designed to improve medication safety in this population [33]. They found that two smartphone applications were successful in identifying relevant medication discrepancies and reducing the number of ADRs. The application which required a higher degree of patient interaction, seemed to do better, including a 60% rate reduction in discrepancies that could seriously harm patients, than the application that required less interaction from the patient. The authors concluded that the application that required a higher degree of engagement was more successful because it stressed the importance of the role of the patient in their own care. They also posited that it opened up communication between the patient and their caregiver and a lack of communication has been reported to be potentially responsible for a significant number of preventable ADRs [34].

Other applications of technology are to develop self-management systems. Self-management support systems have been useful tools for patients with kidney disease as they are able to have better control of their care and daily activities [35]. A study conducted in Toronto examined utilization of a smart phone based system for CKD patients with stage 4 and 5 CKD. The system targeted four behavioral components of self-management, including blood pressure, medication management, symptom assessment, and tracking laboratory results. The findings indicated that patients with high adherence in utilizing the system felt more empowered and reported better control of their health [36].

The emotional experience of the user is also an important factor in the enhancement and promotion of technology use. As an example, the design of the user interface has proven to be significant in predicting patient engagement [37].

CKD patients may be more open to using self-management support systems when they had the freedom to choose whether to use the system and felt the system was safe and easy to use [37].

Improving Technology Acceptance

While there is scant data on strategies to improve technology acceptance, the key factors seem to be ease of use and perceived benefit. As technology is increasingly becoming a part of our patients' daily lives, it is important to develop strategies that encourage them to use it and incorporate it into their healthcare. Those who are unable to use technology can be negatively impacted, as they are more likely to depend on others and experience social isolation. Technology can be particularly beneficial in healthcare settings for the elderly with chronic medical conditions as it can promote independence through increased self-management, monitoring, medication management, and adherence to daily treatment protocols and fluid and dietary restrictions [38]. Being able to use technology such as smart phones, laptops, computers, and tablets as well as patient portals or healthcare systems will allow patients to receive educational materials, information about new resources and/or support in their treatment facility and appointment reminders/cancelations notices [38]. In order to increase older patients' computer self-efficacy and reduce computer anxiety, providers in healthcare settings can offer trainings to teach them how to use the system and when to use specific features. Offering information technology support on an ongoing basis might also increase and improve their utilization. Older patients are more likely to use a technology when they are educated on its usefulness, and how it promotes independence in their lives and when they know and understand how to utilize it [39]. Figure 5.1 presents a conceptual model of how the technology adoption model may be applied to patients with CKD. It highlights the key role that demographic and psychological variables play in driving the two main factors in predicting novel technology adoption; perceived ease of using the technology and its perceived potential benefit.

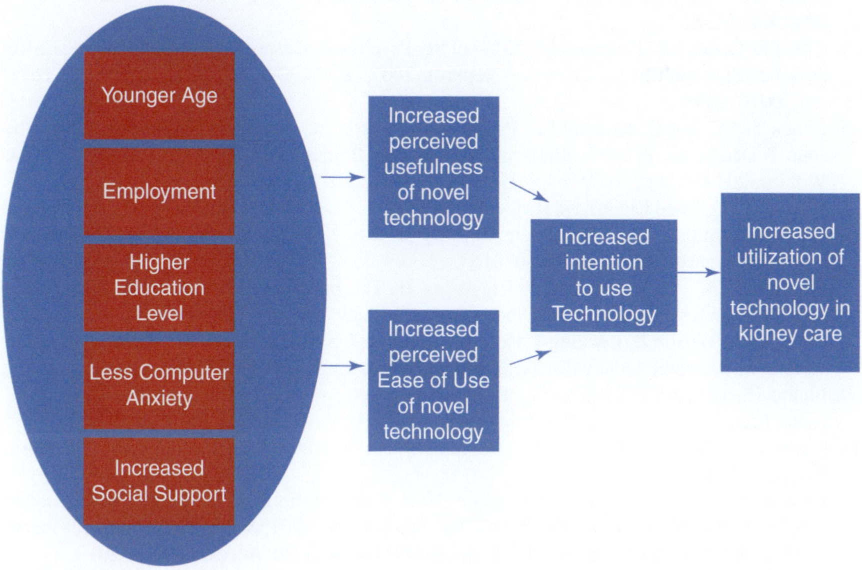

Fig. 5.1 An application of the technology acceptance model in patients with kidney disease

Conclusion

Human response can explain an individual's psychological reactions to their illness, and the types of self-management behaviors they choose to engage in. An understanding of the patient's perception of the demands of the illness and its treatments will allow the clinical team to predict, and possibly preemptively address, some of the additional challenges of patients with CKD. Interventions designed to identify, prevent, and treat depression and anxiety, as well interventions designed to promote engagement in care and novel technologies need to be incorporated into care models for patients with CKD in order to improve treatment and outcome.

References

1. Selye H. Stress in health and disease. Butterworths; 1976. https://books.google.com/books?hl=en&lr=&id=wrfYBAAAQBAJ&oi=fnd&pg=PP1&dq=selye+stress&ots=_jqqtfb8i9&sig=8WMmYlWY40x0QwohBesWe6vpHhw#v=onepage&q=selye%20stress&f=false. Accessed 9 Oct 2019.
2. McEwen BS. Allostasis and allostatic load: implications for neuropsychopharmacology. Neuropsychopharmacology. 2000;22(2):108–24. https://doi.org/10.1016/S0893-133X(99)00129-3.
3. Goldstein DS, McEwen B. Allostasis, homeostats, and the nature of stress. Stress. 2002;5(1):55–8.
4. Cukor D, Cohen SD, Peterson RA, Kimmel PL. Psychosocial aspects of chronic disease: ESRD as a paradigmatic illness. J Am Soc Nephrol. 2007;18(12):3042–55. https://doi.org/10.1681/asn.2007030345.
5. Cohen SD, Cukor D, Kimmel PL. Psychosocial issues. In: Handbook of dialysis. 5th ed; by John T. Daugirdas, Peter G. Blake and Todd S. Ing. Philadelphia, PA: Lippincott Williams & Wilkins, 2014, 900 pp. (ISBN-13: 978-1451144291). (2015): 609–10.
6. Weisbord SD, Fried LF, Arnold RM, et al. Prevalence, severity, and importance of physical and emotional symptoms in chronic hemodialysis patients. J Am Soc Nephrol. 2005;16:2487–94. https://doi.org/10.1681/ASN.2005020157.
7. Murtagh FEM, Addington-Hall J, Higginson IJ. The prevalence of symptoms in end-stage renal disease: a systematic review. Adv Chronic Kidney Dis. 2007;14(1):82–99.
8. Harwood L, Wilson B, Locking-Cusolito H, Sontrop J, Spittal J. Stressors and coping in individuals with chronic kidney disease. Nephrol Nurs J. 2009;36(3):265–301.
9. Flythe JE, Hilliard T, Castillo G, et al. Symptom prioritization among adults receiving in-center hemodialysis: a mixed methods study. Clin J Am Soc Nephrol. 2018;13(5):735–45.
10. Coyne JC, Aldwin C, Lazarus RS. Depression and coping in stressful episodes. J Abnorm Psychol. 1981;90(5):439.
11. Beck A. Cognitive therapy of depression. New York: Guilford; 1979. https://books.google.com/books?hl=en&lr=&id=L09cRS0xWj0C&oi=fnd&pg=PP15&dq=beck+cognitive+therapy&ots=FXPiaJfodn&sig=zeelFzOyirYTRx1hxz841WWHVR0. Accessed 9 Apr 2019.
12. Cukor D, Coplan J, Brown C, et al. Depression and anxiety in urban hemodialysis patients. Clin J Am Soc Nephrol. 2007;2(3):484–90.
13. Kimmel PL, Cukor D, Cohen SD, Peterson RA. Depression in end-stage renal disease patients: a critical review. Adv Chronic Kidney Dis. 2007;14(4):328–34. https://doi.org/10.1053/j.ackd.2007.07.007.

14. Maier SF, Seligman ME. Learned helplessness: theory and evidence. J Exp Psychol Gen. 1976;105(1):3.
15. Khan A, Khan AH, Adnan AS, Sulaiman SAS, Mushtaq S. Prevalence and predictors of depression among hemodialysis patients: a prospective follow-up study. BMC Public Health. 2019;19(1):1–13.
16. Hasin DS, Sarvet AL, Meyers JL, et al. Epidemiology of adult DSM-5 major depressive disorder and its specifiers in the United States. JAMA Psychiat. 2018;75(4):336–46.
17. Zalai D, Szeifert L, Novak M. Psychological distress and depression in patients with chronic kidney disease. In: Seminars in dialysis, vol. 25. Wiley Online Library; 2012. p. 428–38.
18. Schouten RW, Haverkamp GL, Loosman WL, et al. Anxiety symptoms, mortality, and hospitalization in patients receiving maintenance dialysis: a cohort study. Am J Kidney Dis. 2019;74(2):158–66.
19. Kimmel PL, Cukor D. Anxiety symptoms in patients treated with hemodialysis: measurement and meaning. Am J Kidney Dis. 2019;74(2):145–7.
20. Feroze U, Martin D, Kalantar-Zadeh K, Kim JC, Reina-Patton A, Kopple JD. Anxiety and depression in maintenance dialysis patients: preliminary data of a cross-sectional study and brief literature review. J Ren Nutr. 2012;22(1):207–10.
21. de Brito DCS, Machado EL, Reis IA, de Carmo F do LP, Cherchiglia ML. Depression and anxiety among patients undergoing dialysis and kidney transplantation: a cross-sectional study. Sao Paulo Med J. 2019;137(2):137–47.
22. Cukor D, Coplan J, Brown C, et al. Anxiety disorders in adults treated by hemodialysis: a single-center study. Am J Kidney Dis. 2008;52(1):128–36. https://doi.org/10.1053/j.ajkd.2008.02.300.
23. Hedayati SS, Grambow SC, Szczech LA, Stechuchak KM, Allen AS, Bosworth HB. Physician-diagnosed depression as a correlate of hospitalizations in patients receiving long-term hemodialysis. Am J Kidney Dis. 2005;46(4):642–9.
24. Mapes DL, Bragg-Gresham JL, Bommer J, et al. Health-related quality of life in the dialysis outcomes and practice patterns study (DOPPS). Am J Kidney Dis. 2004;44:54–60.
25. Nair D, Cavanaugh KL. Measuring patient activation as part of kidney disease policy: are we there yet? J Am Soc Nephrol. 2020;31(7):1435–43.
26. National Center for Health Statistics, US, 2016. Health, United States, 2015: With special feature on racial and ethnic health disparities.
27. Howard G, Prineas R, Moy C, Cushman M, Kellum M, Temple E, Graham A and Howard V, 2006. Racial and geographic differences in awareness, treatment, and control of hypertension: the REasons for Geographic And Racial Differences in Stroke study. Stroke, 37(5), pp.1171–78.
28. Lee Y, Kozar KA, Larsen KRT. The technology acceptance model: past, present, and future. Commun Assoc Inf Syst. 2003;12(1):50.
29. Czaja SJ, Charness N, Fisk AD, et al. Factors predicting the use of technology: findings from the Center for Research and Education on Aging and Technology Enhancement (CREATE). Psychol Aging. 2006;21(2):333.
30. Dhagarra D, Goswami M, Kumar G. Impact of trust and privacy concerns on technology acceptance in healthcare: an Indian perspective. Int J Med Inform. 2020;141:104164.
31. Hussein WF, Bennett PN, Pace S, et al. The mobile health readiness of people receiving in-center hemodialysis and home dialysis. Clin J Am Soc Nephrol. 2021;16(1):98–106.
32. Laville SM, Gras-Champel V, Moragny J, et al. Adverse drug reactions in patients with CKD. Clin J Am Soc Nephrol. 2020;15(8):1090–102.
33. Ong SW, Jassal SV, Porter EC, et al. Digital applications targeting medication safety in ambulatory high-risk CKD patients: randomized controlled clinical trial. Clin J Am Soc Nephrol. 2021;16(4):532–42.
34. Gandhi TK, Weingart SN, Borus J, et al. Adverse drug events in ambulatory care. N Engl J Med. 2003;348(16):1556–64.

35. Curtin RB, Walters BAJ, Schatell D, Pennell P, Wise M, Klicko K. Self-efficacy and self-management behaviors in patients with chronic kidney disease. Adv Chronic Kidney Dis. 2008;15(2):191–205.
36. Ong SW, Jassal SV, Miller JA, et al. Integrating a smartphone-based self-management system into usual care of advanced CKD. Clin J Am Soc Nephrol. 2016;11(6):1054–62.
37. Wang W, van Lint CL, Brinkman W-P, et al. Renal transplant patient acceptance of a self-management support system. BMC Med Inform Decis Mak. 2017;17(1):1–11.
38. Bonner A, Gillespie K, Campbell KL, et al. Evaluating the prevalence and opportunity for technology use in chronic kidney disease patients: a cross-sectional study. BMC Nephrol. 2018;19(1):1–8.
39. Portz JD, Bayliss EA, Bull S, et al. Using the technology acceptance model to explore user experience, intent to use, and use behavior of a patient portal among older adults with multiple chronic conditions: descriptive qualitative study. J Med Internet Res. 2019;21(4):e11604.

Chapter 6
Current Dietary Advances in Enhancing Adherence in ESRD Patients

Danielle Sobieski and Georgiana Mitrus

General Dietary Guidelines for End Stage Renal Disease Patients

Nutrition therapy and medical treatment go hand in hand toward improving a patient's health; nutrition therapy plays an important supportive measure to facilitate effective medical treatment, and, at the same time, a positive response to nutrition therapy requires successful medical treatment of the underlying disease [1]. It is thought that inflammation and malnutrition are pathophysiologically linked in CKD due to inflammation-induced muscle proteolysis and catabolism. Additionally, pro-inflammatory markers lead to decreased nutrient intake (e.g., depression and decreased appetite), decreased protein synthesis, increased protein catabolism, and increased metabolic rate [2, 3]. In the face of inflammation, nutrition interventions may not be as effective, which increases the risk of malnutrition. Finally, malnutrition may compromise the clinical response to therapy, and the circle continues [1].

The primary role of the registered dietitian in the dialysis setting is to optimize a patient's nutritional status, minimize adverse clinical outcomes, slow the progression of the disease and prevent or treat malnutrition [1]. In this section, we discuss current dietary recommendations to optimize a dialysis patient's nutrition status and prevent malnutrition.

The updated 2020 guidelines from the National Kidney Foundation (NKF) Kidney Disease Outcome Quality (KDOQI) and American of Nutrition and Dietetics (AND) contain several changes from the 2000 guidelines. Please refer to the full report for the extensive guidelines, rationale and ratings of the evidence, recommendations, considerations, and limitations especially in regard to anthropometric and body composition measurements.

D. Sobieski (✉) · G. Mitrus
Danielle Sobieski Nutrition PLLC, Brooklyn, NY, USA

S. J. Saggi, M. O. Salifu (eds.), *Technological Advances in Care of Patients with Kidney Diseases*, https://doi.org/10.1007/978-3-031-11942-2_6

The updated guidelines recommend relying more on clinical judgment, especially when assessing weight and the appropriate weight (Ideal Body Weight, Standard Body Weight, Actual Body Weight, etc.) to use when determining energy needs via resting energy expenditure equations, when indirect calorimetry cannot be used. The guidelines recommend at least monthly weights, BMI (with heights measured periodically) and body composition assessments (e.g., Bioelectrical Impedance, Dual-Energy X-ray Absorptiometry if available) as well as skin fold thickness, waist circumference, conicity index, and/or creatinine kinetics when appropriate, while taking edema and or protein or creatinine supplementation intake into account. The guidelines also include a recommendation that a modified Subjective Global Assessment (SGA), assessing the loss of subcutaneous fat, muscle wasting, and edema, be performed every 6 months. It is suggested that underweight or morbid obesity status based on BMI can be used as a predictor of higher mortality, while overweight or obesity status based on BMI can be used as a predictor of lower morality, unless the patient is 65 years or older (however, this association between weight status and mortality has not found to be significant).

When determining malnutrition, BMI alone cannot be used as a diagnosis for malnutrition unless the BMI is less than 18 kg/m^2, however, a better indicator of malnutrition is the percentage change of usual (dry) weight [4]. Also, it is important to note that malnutrition can occur at any BMI, not only with underweight patients. In 2012, The American Society for Parenteral and Enteral Nutrition (ASPEN) put forth malnutrition diagnostic criteria that registered dietitians are specially equipped to determine if the patient meets two of the six criteria needed to diagnose malnutrition (percent weight change included) [5]. For the purpose of this chapter we outlined the updated guidelines for calories, protein, sodium, phosphorus, calcium, and potassium in Tables 6.1 and 6.2.

Table 6.1 Updated guidelines for protein, energy, and electrolytes for clinically stable dialysis patients

	HD	PD
Protein g/kg[a,b]	1.0–1.2 stable (consider higher levels for diabetic or acutely ill)	1.0–1.2 stable (consider higher levels for diabetic or acutely ill)
Energy kcal/kg[b]	30–35	30–35 Including dialysate
Sodium mg/day[c]	<2300	2000; monitor fluid balance
Potassium mEq/day	Maintain serum potassium WNL	Maintain serum potassium WNL
Fiber g/day	20–25	20–25
Fluids cc/day	750–1500; ensure sodium balance	Maintain balance

Table 6.1 (continued)

	HD	PD
Calcium mg/day[d]	≤1000; maintain serum calcium WNL	800; maintain serum calcium WNL
Phosphorus mg/day[e]	Individualized needs; maintain serum phosphorus WNL	Individualized needs; maintain serum phosphorus WNL

Adapted from National Kidney Foundation, *Pocket guide to nutritional assessment of the patient with chronic kidney disease, fifth edition* [6], and Updated with information from KDOQI 2020
Additional References: Kopple et al. [7]; NKF K/DOQI Clinical practice guidelines for nutrition in chronic renal failure [8]; KDIGO CKD Work Group [9]
Note: Biomarkers such as nPCR, serum albumin, or serum prealbumin can be considered complementary tools to assess nutritional status but cannot be used in isolation to assess nutritional status
[a] The recommendations for a particular type of protein are divided. There are studies suggesting protein recommendations of at least 50% high biological value (HBV) (nitrogen incorporated into the body/total absorbed nitrogen >75%), such as proteins in eggs, fish, poultry, meat, and dairy products, which contain essential amino acids [10], while latest KDOQI 2020 opinion alleges "inadequate evidence to recommend a particular protein type (plant vs animal) in terms of the effects on nutritional status, calcium or phosphorus levels, or the blood lipid profile." Patients are usually in a negative protein balance if their intake is restricted to less than 0.5 g protein/kg/day unless they are provided with essential AA supplementation [11]. Patients who are at risk of hyper- and/or hypoglycemia may need higher levels of dietary protein intake to maintain glycemic control [4]
[b] Use estimated dry weight. For obese patients, calculate the adjusted body weight from the ideal body weight plus 25% of the excess weight. Clinical judgment should be used to determine the method to assess and decide which "weight" to use in predictive equations if indirect calorimetry is not used
[c] While strict sodium control may be more difficult in an outpatient setting, evidence suggests that sodium control alone may be more powerful than fluid restriction on maintaining stable weight [12]. It is recommended to limit sodium in order to reduce blood pressure and improve volume control (KDOQI 2020)
[d] May adjust calcium intake (dietary calcium, calcium supplements or calcium-based binders) with consideration of concurrent use of vitamin D analogs and calcimimetics in order to avoid hypercalcemia (KDOQI 2020)
[e] It is reasonable to consider the source. Organic phosphorus from both animal and plant foods has an intestinal absorption rate of only 40–60%. Alternatively, inorganic phosphorus, such as phosphates added to foods during processing, has an absorption rate of greater than 90% [13]. It is recommended to adjust dietary phosphorus intake to maintain serum phosphate levels in the normal range (KDOQI 2020)

Table 6.2 Daily vitamin supplementation for CKD

Vitamins	RDA	HD	PD
Ascorbic acid mg/day	75–90	RDA	RDA
B1 (Thiamine) mg/day	1.1–1.2	RDA	RDA
B2 (Riboflavin) mg/day	1.1–1.3	RDA	RDA
B6 (Pyridoxamine) mg/day	1.3–1.7	10	10
B12 (Cobalamin) µg/day	2.4	RDA	RDA

(continued)

Table 6.2 (continued)

Vitamins	RDA	HD	PD
Biotin μg/day	30	RDA	RDA
Folic acid mg/day	0.400	1	1
Niacin mg/day	14–16	RDA	RDA
Pantothenic acid mg/day	5	RDA	RDA
Vitamin A μg RE/day	700–900	None	None
25-hydroxy vitamin D IU	600	[a]	[a]
Vitamin E (IU)	22.5	15	Up to RDA
Vitamin K μg/day	90–120	With antibiotic therapy, 10 mg/day	With antibiotic therapy, 10 mg/day

Adapted from National Kidney Foundation, *Pocket guide to nutritional assessment of the patient with chronic kidney disease, fifth edition* [6], and updated with information from KDOQI 2020
RDA recommended dietary allowance
[a] Consider supplementation to correct deficiency (<30 mmol/L) with Vitamin D3 (cholecalciferol), Vitamin D2 (ergocalciferol) or other Vitamin D analogs, while maintaining PTH and calcium balance

Where Can End Stage Renal Disease Patients Find Pertinent Nutrition Information

Registered Dietitians at dialysis centers will likely have patient education handouts readily available. However, to further motivate patients to take a proactive role in their care, we encourage patients to find accurate and credible information on their own [14]. Patients should feel competent and empowered to do their own research to expand their knowledge of renal nutrition and in doing so encourage self-management [15]. However, this can prove to be more daunting than expected, for example, as a study by Lambert et al. concluded that only 18% of YouTube videos and 73% of websites were considered accurate and, in a study researching available phone applications, only 50% contained accurate information, consistent with evidence-based guidelines [14]. It is therefore imperative to first teach patients how to avoid nutrition misinformation (i.e., fads, fraud, and misdirected claims) [16].

We recommend teaching patients how to look for reliable resources Table 6.3 and what to avoid Table 6.4 [16, 17].

Another trap that patients may fall into, and which can be especially distressing to renal patients are food marketing misconceptions. On top of having to follow a more difficult diet pattern, patients are bombarded by potential buzzwords like natural, processed, organic. It is important to educate on these terms to lessen the confusion around them and help patients make their best food decisions [18]. Table 6.5 lists common food marketing misconceptions [18].

From here we can discuss what kind of diet pattern and foods matter most to the patient, review their laboratory work with them and figure out which foods and electrolytes to adjust to better serve their health. Some great sites to find reliable

Table 6.3 What to look for when searching for reliable nutrition information

• Websites with .edu, .org, or .gov, consider eatright.org
• Review author's qualifications
• Look for cited and current sources (for example, for sources within the last 5 years)

Table 6.4 Common red flags

• Resources promising "quick fixes"
• Resources that are seemingly too good to be true
• Lists of "good" and "bad" foods
• Oversimplified claims, claims made based on single study, or claims with research "currently underway"
• Resources that include non-science-based testimonials
• Resources created by unlicensed or uncredentialed professionals

Table 6.5 Common food marketing misconceptions

Term	Meaning
Natural	No formal definition, but typically used on foods that contain no artificial ingredients or added colors
Whole	No formal definition, but typically thought of as not processed or minimally processed or refined and do not have added ingredients and close to its original form
Processed	Typically misunderstood, processed has been equated to meaning that a food is "bad," but in reality, it means the food went through a change in character (e.g., raw nuts vs roasted nuts)
Local	No definitive distance range
Organic	• Has a specific and legal meaning by the USDA • Meat, poultry, eggs, and dairy are from animals that are not given antibiotics or growth hormones • Plant foods are produced without using most conventional pesticides, fertilizers made with synthetic ingredients or sewage sludge, bioengineering or ionizing radiation. • Farms are inspected by a government approved certifier • Common organic labels – "100% organic" – "Organic" at least 95% ingredients – "Made with organic ingredients" at least 70% ingredients

nutrition information are listed in Table 6.6. In particular, The American Kidney Fund organization has great modern and complete information and recipes that are free to download and print. Competency in reading nutrition labels is very important for patients, if possible and not inhibited by age, literacy level, poor eyesight, or language barriers, etc. The Renal Dietetics Practice Group has a great "*Nutrition*

Table 6.6 Additional helpful nutrition information sites for patients

• American kidney fund: Kidney friendly diet: https://www.kidneyfund.org/kidney-disease/chronic-kidney-disease-ckd/kidney-friendly-diet-for-ckd.html
• American kidney fund: Kidney kitchen: https://kitchen.kidneyfund.org/ [great downloads]
• National Kidney Foundation: https://www.kidney.org/nutrition/Dialysis
• American Association of Kidney Patients: https://aakp.org/center-for-patient-research-and-education/kidney-friendly-recipes/ [links to support groups]
• Dialysis patient citizens: https://www.dialysispatients.org
• Kidney school: https://kidneyschool.org
• Renal support network: https://www.rsnhope.org

Facts Label" handout. It explains what and where to look for the most pertinent information and explains the information in a way that is helpful for patients. The handout also reviews what ingredients to search for when looking for hidden sources of sodium, potassium, and phosphorus. Members of the Renal Dietetics Group also have access to a comprehensive handout by the group, "*Resources for Eating Well: For Chronic Kidney Disease or Dialysis.*" This handout includes websites, cookbooks, apps, delivered meals, and meal planning services for patients.

Mobile applications have a huge potential to increase nutrition knowledge, decrease non-adherence, and increase positive health outcomes via engaging and encouraging patient self-management [18, 19]. However, at this time there is no single renal nutrition application that is recommended for all dialysis patients due to the complex nature of the disease, the patient's comorbidities, and the patient's individual needs that change over time [15]. Applications like MyFitnessPal may be helpful for some tech-savvy patients who enjoy using apps to track or find nutrition information but should be used carefully and in conjunction with medical nutrition therapy and counseling to ensure that the correct information is being provided. Remembering to take and consume medications such as phosphate binders or calcium supplements may be improved by applications such as Medisafe, and in doing so would help maintain a patient's laboratory values and further reduce food restrictions. More on mobile applications in the next section.

Planning Kidney Friendly Meals

It is important for patients to be aware of and up to date with their monthly nutrition labs, and understand that what they eat has an accumulative effect; considering the limitations of dialysis on removing phosphorus and potassium [a typical dialysis treatment removes 70–100 mEq (210–300 mEq/week for patients on thrice weekly HD) and 350 mg of phosphorus], if patients (with typically high serum potassium) consume high potassium foods throughout the month, their potassium lab value will likely be high, even though a patient might restrict potassium a day or two before treatment. Once patients become aware of this fact, a plan with the registered dietitian regarding what electrolytes and macronutrients to adjust may be started. Below is a step-by-step list of how to plan meals. Planning meals can be time consuming but will become easier as time progresses. It is important to note that this may not be easily possible for some patients, such as those with depression, mobile disability, poor eyesight, cognitive decline or on food stamps, without some adjustments.

1. Help the patient/caregiver understand their labs and discuss with the patient/caregiver what to focus on for the next month or agreed upon time frame (maybe food related or something else if there are more pressing issues).
2. Help the patient review recipes online or from cookbooks (there are a lot of kidney friendly cookbooks available for free if needed). Adjust the recipe to suit the patient's nutrition needs.
3. Encourage the patient's family, friends or caregivers to be involved if possible. Reminder—just because a recipe may be "kidney friendly" does not mean someone else cannot or would not want to eat it (unless they have abnormal labs).
4. Encourage the patient/caregiver to take inventory of what they already have in their pantry or refrigerator. Then, with the recipes, start writing down a shopping list (there are some general renal friendly grocery lists available if needed). Meal planning would be a great activity to do during dialysis.
5. Next, the patient/caregiver is ready to go to the grocery store, shop online, or the food pantry at a planned time and preferably when they are not hungry.
6. Lastly, patients or caregivers should be mindful (if possible) of reviewing nutrition labels for trans fats, added sugars, calcium, potassium and phosphorus. The more patients/caregivers do this, the more comfortable they will become with nutrition labels and the less time grocery shopping will take.

If the patient is on food stamps, has a strict budget and/or relies on food pantries, or receives hot meals from a meal program, the provider should work with the social worker to ensure the patient is using all the resources available for proper nutrition. While it is possible to eat healthy and follow most recommendations on a strict budget, monetary barriers will likely require more time planning and prepping meals, and extra help may be needed. If a patient has their food prepared by family, friends or a caregiver, they will need to be involved in learning about kidney nutrition and in understanding the recommendations provided by the dialysis team. For patients with depression, cognitive dysfunction or decline, additional help may be required. Meal prepping can be overwhelming and time consuming and can be very difficult to initiate and carry out.

As for building a healthy meal, the plate method is a helpful technique that can be used to manage macronutrients, carbohydrate intake, as well as aid with weight management. It involves dividing the plate to enable measuring out appropriate portion sizes of different foods. For dialysis patients it is recommended that a quarter of the plate is filled with protein rich food, a quarter of the plate with grains or starchy vegetables, and the remaining half the plate with fruits and vegetables. The food options on the plate should be adjusted based on the patient's electrolyte laboratory values, as well as individual protein and energy needs. The recommended fluid allowance should be adjusted based on fluid status. Patients should be encouraged to take binders as prescribed (before, during, and/or after meals, as per prescription or team instructions). A mobile application or alarm clock may serve as a helpful reminder.

How to Help Patients Achieve Recommended Nutrition Goals

As the KDOQI Guidelines state, during nutrition assessments it is imperative that the registered dietitian assesses factors beyond dietary intake (e.g., medication use, knowledge, beliefs, attitudes, behavior, access to food, depression, cognitive function) to effectively plan interventions [4]. Additional factors seemingly unrelated to nutrition need to be dealt with in order for recommendations to work. For example, patients unable to pay for food or medications will be unlikely to keep their nutrition related labs within normal limits and are therefore at increased risk for malnutrition. Or a patient with severe depression or cognitive dysfunction will be unlikely to be able to carry out recommendations that involve multiple steps and planning, and may need additional help from caregivers. A multidisciplinary approach and having respect from the healthcare team is vital to our patient's overall health. When barriers that patients face can be reduced, patients are better equipped to meet their health and nutrition related goals.

Building a good rapport and maintaining an open dialog with the patient is equally important when providing effective nutrition counseling ("a supportive process to set priorities, establish goals, and create individualized action plans that acknowledge and foster responsibility for self-care") and patient-centered care [20]. Effective nutrition counseling is a collaborative endeavor between provider and patient, in order to determine what goals are achievable for the patient, and how the provider can offer choices, enabling the patient to reach their goals. Counseling certainly includes education, but active listening is more effective than providing handouts or education that may not be helpful to a patient that may be distracted by non-nutrition related barriers. Nutrition counseling takes several counseling theories and strategies into account, finding ways to better communicate such as listening more, asking more open-ended questions, avoiding conversation blockers ("you should," "you need to," etc.), as well as building confidence when ending conversations.

Motivational interviewing (MI) has been shown to promote adherence and improve well-being in kidney patients. Miller and Rollnick define MI as "a collaborative, goal-oriented style of communication with a particular attention to the language of change. It is designed to strengthen personal motivation for and commitment to a specific goal by eliciting and exploring the person's own reasons for change within an atmosphere of acceptance and compassion [21]. MI focuses on "working together with patients in a partnership, accepting the patients' stance in treatment, compassionately promoting the patients' welfare, and evoking from patients their strengths and resources that would help them change." In conversation with the patient, "the provider draws out the patients' arguments that favor change (called "change talk"), while understanding and helping to resolve, as needed, arguments that sustain unhealthy behavior (called "sustain talk")," in such a way that patients talk themselves into making changes [22].

Once the desire to elicit change has been instilled in the ESRD patient, the provider can provide the patient with different learning experiences and find different ways to educate, by using/creating handouts, reviewing tech-based applications, bulletin boards, programs, newsletters, social media, and support groups as a way to educate without overloading patients with too much education [23]. Simple tactics such as setting medication alarms or having paper or magnet reminders on pantry or refrigerator doors are easy to create and may help some patients who require simpler or non-electronic educational tools to take their medication or limit a certain food.

It is entirely reasonable to consider creating more and better applications for dialysis patients since mobile applications can reach many people with different ages and socioeconomic status' [14, 24]. Thoughtful applications should empower motivated patients to take a proactive role in their health, navigate challenges, support recommendations, and improve communication and engagement between patient and healthcare team to promote positive health outcomes [14, 25]. Unfortunately, at this time, a lot of mobile applications for renal patients are missing the mark. Less than half of renal mobile applications were found to contain accurate information, and more were found to have poor design or be inappropriate for patients with inadequate health literacy; most applications also were found to have errors in nutrition data [14], lack of verified reviews or support by reputable organizations [19, 26], privacy issues, and a lack of personalization [26].

Moving forward, we need more registered dietitians along with members of the multidisciplinary team to create mobile applications for renal patients [14]. App creators should take into account: patient perception and usefulness vs the content quality and security of the information and design, figure out how to reduce lack of confidence and frustration with app-based tech design, create ways to improve communications between patient, caregiver, friends and family, and provide real time data review [14, 15, 24, 27]. At present, time health providers are limited to providing patients with continuously reviewed apps and websites and ask for patient's feedback; an app preferred by the patient is more likely to encourage healthy eating behaviors and promote nutritional well-being.

What Exists and What Needs to Improve to Help ESRD Patients Meet Their Nutrition Goals

Not only does kidney disease come with its own unique set of challenges, but also each patient is unique, requiring individualized nutrition interventions. Unfortunately, there is no single site, handout or mobile application that can serve as a one-stop-shop for information. Certain dialysis websites provide nutrition related newsletters, support groups and other programs, and even social media accounts to provide information catered to their site; each source, however, is different and is limited in the amount of information it provides.

The ESRD patient is highly unique, as is the disease. Patients require lifelong learning of their condition, and interventions they can utilize, with the help of a registered dietitian or appropriate team member, to improve their nutrition quality of life. In doing so, providers may want to move away from using words such as "non-compliance," "non-adherence," "strict," and "control" when discussing with patients. Providers must be on the patients' team and understand that their quality of life, or the quality of life they want for themselves, is what is most important. No one is perfect, nor do they need to be, but if patients are set up for success and want to feel better, they likely can achieve that most of the time, by following individualized nutrition recommendations in conjunction with the counsel of the multidisciplinary team.

In this chapter, we have discussed the importance of medical nutrition therapy in end stage renal disease, provided information on the updated guidelines, how and where to find good, reliable information, how to plan nutrition goals and recommendations, how to create effective interventions, as well as ideas on how to better use app-based technology for ESRD patients. Most importantly, we want to emphasize the crucial cooperation between the healthcare team, working together and providing patient-centered care, as providing the most benefit; nutrition has a pivotal support role to medical interventions, and medical interventions are increasingly more effective in a patient who is nutritionally optimized.

References

1. ASPEN (2020) Adult malnutrition: frequently asked questions. Malnutrition Solution Center, Addition Resources/Publications. http://www.nutritioncare.org/malnutrition/; file:///Users/daniellesobieski/Downloads/AMN%20FAQs%20November%202014_Final.pdf. Accessed 23 Mar 2018.
2. Kirkland LL, Kashiwagi DT, Brantley S, Scheurer D, Varkey P. Nutrition in the hospitalized patient. J Hosp Med. 2013;8(1):52–8.
3. Weiss AJ, Fingar KR, Barrett ML, Elixhauser A, Steiner CA, Guenter P, Brown MH, Characteristics of hospital stays involving malnutrition. HCUP statistical brief #210. Rockville, MD: Agency for Healthcare Research and Quality; 2013. http://www.hcup-us.ahrq.gov/reports/statbriefs/sb210-Malnutrition-Hospital-Stays-2013.pdf.
4. Ikizler, TA, Burrowes JD, Byham-Gray LD, et al. KDOQI nutrition in CKD guideline work group. KDOQI clinical practice for nutrition in CKD: 2020 update. Am J Kidney Dis. 2020:76(3 suppl 1):S1–107.
5. White JV, Guenter P, Jensen G, Malone A, Schofield M, Academy Malnutrition Work Group; A.S.P.E.N. Board of Directors. Consensus statement: Academy of Nutrition and Dietetics and American Society for parenteral and enteral nutrition: characteristics recommended for the identification and documentation of adult malnutrition (undernutrition). JPEN Parenter Enteral Nutr. 2012;36(3):275–83.
6. National Kidney Foundation (2015) Pocket guide to nutrition assessment, 5th edn. Chapter 4, nutrition prescription.

7. Kopple JD, Massry SG, Kalantar-Zedeh K, editors. Nutritional management of renal disease. 3rd ed. New York: Elsevier Academic Press; 2013.
8. NKF K/DOQI. Clinical practice guidelines for nutrition in chronic renal failure. Am J Kidney Dis. 2000;35(6):S1–S140.
9. KDIGO CKD Work Group. KDIGO 2012 clinical practice guideline for the evaluation and management of chronic kidney disease. Kidney Int. 2013;3(Suppl):S1–S150.
10. Zha Y, Qian Q. Protein nutrition and malnutrition in CKD and ESRD. Nutrients. 2017;9(3):208.
11. Wilcox CS, Tischer CC. Handbook of nephrology and hypertension. 6th ed. Philadelphia: Lippincott Williams & Wilkins; 2008.
12. Tomson CRV. Advising dialysis patients to restrict fluid intake without restricting sodium intake is not based on evidence and is a waste of time. Nephrol Dialysis Transplant. 2001;16(8):1538–42. https://doi.org/10.1093/ndt/16.8.1538.
13. Kalantar-Zadeh K, Gutekunst L, Mehrotra R, et al. Understanding sources of dietary phosphorus in the treatment of patients with chronic kidney disease. Clin J Am Soc Nephrol. 2010;5:519–30.
14. Lambert K, et al. Should we recommend renal diet–related apps to our patients? An evaluation of the quality and health literacy demand of renal diet–related mobile applications. J Ren Nutr. 2017;27(6):430–8. https://doi.org/10.1053/j.jrn.2017.06.007.
15. Kosa SD, et al. Nutritional mobile applications for CKD patients: systematic review. Kidney Int Rep. 2019;4(3):399–407. https://doi.org/10.1016/j.ekir.2018.11.016.
16. Bellows L, Moore R. Nutrition misinformation: how to identify fraud and misleading claims. Colorado State University Extension; 2013. https://extension.colostate.edu/topic-areas/nutrition-food-safety-health/nutrition-misinformation-how-to-identify-fraud-and-misleading-claims-9-350/#top. Accessed 4 Apr 2020.
17. U.S. Food and Drug Administration, Office of Regulatory Affairs. Health fraud scams. FDA; 2020. www.fda.gov/consumers/health-fraud-scams. Accessed 4 Apr 2020.
18. Klemm S. Understanding food marketing terms. EatRight; 2019. www.eatright.org/food/nutrition/nutrition-facts-and-food-labels/understanding-food-markting-terms. Accessed 4 April 2020.
19. Siddique AB, et al. Mobile apps for the care management of chronic kidney and end-stage renal diseases: systematic search in app stores and evaluation. JMIR MHealth UHealth. 2019;7(9):e12604. https://doi.org/10.2196/12604.
20. American Dietetic Association Evidence Analysis Library. Nutrition counseling evidence analysis project; 2020. https://www.andeal.org/topic.cfm?menu=315. Accessed 18 Dec 2020.
21. Miller W, Rollnick S. Motivational interviewing: facilitating change. 3rd ed. New York: The Guilford Press; 2012.
22. Sanders KA, Whited A, Martino S. Motivational interviewing for patients with chronic kidney disease. Semin Dial. 2013;26(2):175–9.
23. Hunt K. A clinical guide to nutrition care in kidney disease, 2nd ed. Appendix B counseling skills for the renal dietitian. Academy of Nutrition and Dietetics; 2013. p. 275–2770.
24. Singh K, et al. Patients' and nephrologists' evaluation of patient-facing smartphone apps for CKD. Clin J Am Soc Nephrol. 2019;14(4):523–29. https://doi.org/10.2215/cjn.10370818.
25. Zanetti-Yabur A, et al. Exploring the usage of a mobile phone application in transplanted patients to encourage medication compliance and education. Am J Surg. 2017;214(4):743–7. https://doi.org/10.1016/j.amjsurg.2017.01.026.
26. Topf JM, Swapnil H. Got CKD? There's an app for that! Clin J Am Soc Nephrol. 2019;14(4):491–2. https://doi.org/10.2215/cjn.02350219.
27. Sarkar U, et al. Usability of commercially available mobile applications for diverse patients. J Gen Intern Med. 2016;31(12):1417–26. https://doi.org/10.1007/s11606-016-3771-6.

Chapter 7
Current Strategies to Enhance Opportunities for Patients with End Stage Kidney Disease to Receive a Kidney Transplant

Sarthak Virmani and Richard Formica

Kidney transplantation is the best treatment for most patients with kidney failure progressing to end stage kidney disease (ESKD). It is a long known fact that transplantation reduces the mortality and significantly improves the quality of life of those requiring some form of renal replacement therapy [1] . Occasionally however, medical, surgical, or psychosocial factors preclude kidney transplantation in some patients.

The challenges for a prospective candidate to successfully undergo and enjoy the benefits of a kidney transplant can be broadly divided into pre-transplantation and post-transplantation.

Providing an equal access to organ transplantation to all members of society and ensuring equitable allocation of procured organs from deceased donors remains an ongoing topic of discussion among policy makers in the pre-transplant realm. On the other hand, maintenance of a transplanted allograft's health, and prolonging its lifespan, such that the transplant recipient can enjoy its benefit for the remainder of his or her life, remains the Achilles heel of post-transplant care. In this chapter, we shall briefly discuss some of these challenges, and the strategies patients and their medical provider can adopt to overcome these barriers.

As per the latest Annual Data Report of the Scientific Registry of Transplant Recipients (SRTR), the overall number of kidney transplants in the country have increased steadily since 2015, reaching the highest count of 24,273 in the year 2019 [2]. This is about 24% of the total 101,337 patients on the kidney transplantation waitlist as of December 31, 2019. Unfortunately, an estimated 40% of these listed patients are listed "inactive" on the waitlist and will not be considered for a kidney transplant offer.

S. Virmani (✉) · R. Formica
Section of Nephrology, Department of Medicine, Yale School of Medicine, Yale University, New Haven, CT, USA
e-mail: sarthak.virmani@yale.edu; richard.formica@yale.edu

S. J. Saggi, M. O. Salifu (eds.), *Technological Advances in Care of Patients with Kidney Diseases*, https://doi.org/10.1007/978-3-031-11942-2_7

The most common reason for these patients to remain inactive on the waitlist is the inability to complete the workup required for establishing suitable candidacy. This involves, but is not limited to, age appropriate screening for malignancies, risk stratification of cardiac health, establishing good psychosocial health and support, objective assessment of good overall health and lack of frailty. Historically, this required multiple trips to the transplantation center and a grueling process of keeping tabs of which tests have been performed and which remain outstanding. Current practices have certainly helped overcome some of these logistical barriers. More efficient use of electronic medical records (EMR), easier sharing of records between providers and improved collaboration across different care delivery systems have helped the transplant centers keep track of multitude of studies for each of their patients. HIPPA compliant internal communication between dialysis providers, primary care providers and transplant centers using various EMR messaging tools has certainly expedited the evaluation process. Moreover, EMR use can be optimized to show active reports of listing requirements, identify patients with specific risk factors, blood types, and contribute to equitable and prompt matching of recipients to appropriate organ offers. Patient portals where the patients can view their own progress toward actively being waitlisted, send and receive non-urgent messages to and from their providers, receive reminders for their upcoming appointments are some of the ways EMRs help improve the patient experience as well. Most centers have transitioned to a one-day centralized work up, a one stop shop for a prospective recipient to undergo workup reducing the burden on the patients for multiple trips, time away from work and most importantly, leading to a decreased time from primary evaluation to being actively waitlisted for kidney transplantation [3].

Despite an increasing number of patients being transplanted, there exists a great deal of misinformation regarding kidney transplantation in the community. Primary care providers (PCP), general nephrologists and dialysis personnel play a pivotal role in encouraging and navigating these patients through the kidney transplantation evaluation process which can often seem to be too complex and daunting. A potential recipient's PCP and general nephrologist can ensure that they are up to date with age appropriate malignancy screenings, their comorbidities thoroughly evaluated and well managed, and are in otherwise good health. This certainly expedites the evaluation by the transplantation team and significantly expedites the active listing of a prospective candidate on the deceased donor kidney waitlist.

Late referral to a transplantation center is yet another barrier to kidney transplantation. Although current Organ Procurement and Transplantation Network (OPTN) policy allows for an approved candidate to start accumulating wait time from the time their glomerular filtration rate (GFR), or equivalent measure is $\leq$20 ml/min, often patients are referred to a transplantation center after dialysis is initiated. This leads to loss of precious time during which the prospective recipient could have been evaluated and possibly be offered a pre-emptive kidney transplantation (Fig. 7.1). The paradigm needs to shift from dialysis being a bridge for transplant to undergoing a transplant prior to reaching ESKD requiring dialysis.

Living donor transplantation should certainly be the focus of every transplant candidate. It is associated with a higher probability of immediate allograft function

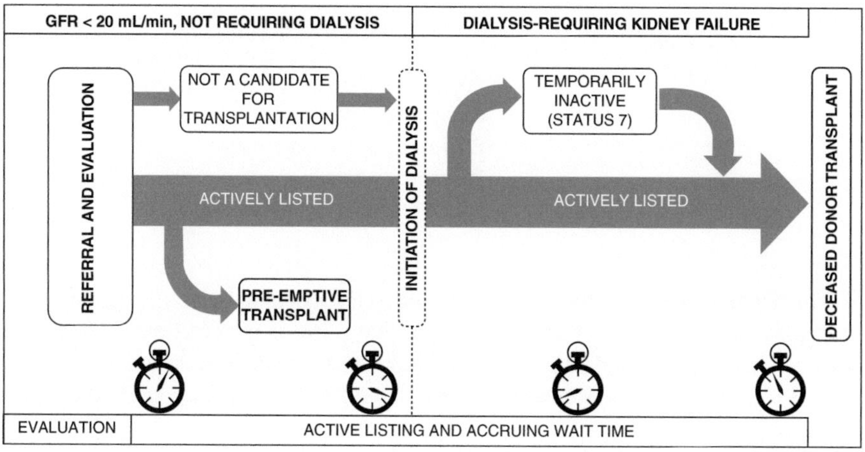

Fig. 7.1 Transplantation evaluation timeline. Note that prospective candidates can start accruing time on the waitlist before the initiation of dialysis. [Image adapted from Virmani S, Asch WS. The Role of the General Nephrologist in Evaluating Patients for Kidney Transplantation: Core Curriculum 2020. Am J Kidney Dis. 2020;76(4):567–79]

and longer allograft survival as compared to a deceased donor kidney transplantation. Some candidates often feel hesitant discussing living donation with friends and family. Although the reason for this hesitancy is often complex and personal, it requires extensive education on the part of the transplantation center to both the prospective recipient and donors regarding the risks and benefits of living donation. Each transplant center adopts practices based on a combination of local resources, surgical and medical expertise and comfort gained from experience with previous patients while evaluating prospective living donors. Social media platforms are also playing an increasing role in prospective recipients initiating these conversations and finding prospective donors online.

Some of the other strategies adopted to improve the patient's chances to receive a kidney transplant include blood type incompatible living donor transplants. Often, prospective living donors are turned away from being evaluated by misinformed community providers or prospective recipients themselves as they are not the exact blood type match. This does not have to be the case. In fact, some donors with blood type A2 are compatible to, and have successfully donated to recipients with blood type B for several years now. Paired exchange programs have played an important role in helping mis-matched pairs as well. Through these, an incompatible donor and recipient pair are jointly introduced into a "swap," with another incompatible but complementary pair.

Although the allocation of procured organs is a complex process involving just and equitable matching of recipients to donors, it is the candidate's kidney allocation score (KAS) that mainly guides this process. Total time accrued on the waitlist is just one of the many factors that contributes to the calculation of this score (Table 7.1), with variable contributions by each factor.

Table 7.1 Candidate factors contributing to the Kidney Allocation Score (KAS) calculation

Factors contributing to the KAS score of a candidate
Qualified time spent waiting on the waitlist
Degree of sensitization (calculated panel reactive antibodies, cPRA)
Prior living organ donor status
Pediatric candidates
HLA-DR mismatch with the donor

The United Network for Organ Sharing (UNOS) and Scientific Registry of Transplant Recipients (SRTR) websites provide a lot of information for patients, non-transplant and transplant providers on how this intricate process works and how various other scoring systems are used for efficient matching and allocation of organs.

Once transplanted, maintenance of good allograft health, protecting it from immune rejection and prolonging its life becomes the main aim of transplant providers and patients alike. The science of transplantation has come a long way from the early 1910s when xenografts procured from dogs, goats, and pigs were implanted in humans. These universally failed within a few days and led to the death of the grafts and patients. Although the first kidney transplantation from one human to another happened in December 1954 [4], with one identical twin donating to the other, it was the introduction of immunosuppressant medications that led to widespread success of allotransplantation. Immunosuppressive medications remain the backbone of preventing immunological activation and damage to these allografts.

Safeguarding the allograft from immunological injury requires walking a tight rope, balancing a state of excess immunosuppression leading to opportunistic infections, and that of less than optimal immunosuppression leading to immune activation and rejection of the graft. While multiple agents and immunosuppressive regimens have been identified over the years, the transplant scientific community is yet to find the best one-size-fits-all recipe of immunosuppressants.

Induction immunosuppression is a combination of anti-rejection medications given at the time of the transplant surgery to prevent early graft rejection. The choice of these medications depends on the risk of rejection in the recipient, which is stratified by the recipients age, degree of sensitization (having pre-formed antibodies against the allograft), and other factors that contribute to immunological risk. It is these risk profiles that guide individualization of the induction regimens to each patient.

Maintenance immunosuppression are anti-rejection medications that are administered for the entire life of the allograft to prevent late immune activation and rejection of the transplant. Prompt initiation of these drugs to rapidly reach therapeutic ranges in the first few days of the transplant are essential to prevent delayed rejections. As each recipient metabolizes these medications differently, the traditional approach to achieving therapeutic range was trial and error based. Current practice includes incorporating precision medicine techniques such as pharmacogenomics to guide this therapy. By studying how genes alter the recipient's response to these medications, we can predict a safe and effective dose much before the patient takes the first dose of these medications, not only reaching target levels sooner but sustaining levels for longer.

Some of the more commonly used maintenance immunosuppression medications (e.g., CNIs, calcineurin inhibitors) are doubled edged swords as they tend to cause scarring and contribute to the subsequent failure of the transplanted kidney. Over the past decade, the transplant community has added newer agents to their armamentarium that avoid the use of CNIs and do not appear to cause kidney scarring thus improving the longevity of the transplanted kidney [5].

Frequent clinic visits and close monitoring of allograft function using various parameters including blood and urine tests, become a part of a kidney transplant recipient's life. While immunotolerance—a state in which the foreign graft does not lead to an immune response in the host, remains the goal of transplantation, newer technologies for early identification of immune activation and risk of rejection have been developed and are now commercially available for use. Although a biopsy of the precious allograft remains the best way to identify a rejection currently, liquid biopsies and non-invasive tests using cell free donor derived DNA and gene expression testing are increasingly being utilized to indicate a deviation from immune quiescence. These relatively new tests promise to capture rejection early leading to early intervention and prolonged graft life.

The future of kidney transplantation is bright. Exciting prospects in the near future include xeno-transplantation (transplantation of organs across different species), wearable artificial kidneys (WAKs), and implantable bio-artificial kidneys (BAKs) [6]. As of recent literature, WAKs are undergoing prime time clinical trials under the supervision of the Food and Drug Administration authority while the rest are still in earlier stages of development or animal trials. While these new devices promise to perform the physical functions of filtration through membranes and sieving out toxic materials from the blood, they come with their own limitations and challenges. Although these devices make dialysis more tolerable and potable, their long-term outcomes and effect on life expectancy of patients requiring kidney replacement therapy remains to be seen. While we work to close the gap between the patients that require long-term dialysis (approximately 750,000 in 2019 per the United States Renal Data System) and the number of patients that receive a transplant in a given year (approximately 24,000 per the 2019 Annual Data Report of the OPTN/SRTR) these devices come with a promise of improving the quality of life of the remainder of the patients that are awaiting a transplantation.

References

1. Schnuelle P, Lorenz D, Trede M, Van Der Woude FJ. Impact of renal cadaveric transplantation on survival in end-stage renal failure: evidence for reduced mortality risk compared with hemodialysis during long-term follow-up. J Am Soc Nephrol. 1998;9:2135–41.
2. Hart A, Lentine KL, Smith JM, Miller JM, Skeans MA, Prentice M, Robinson A, Foutz J, Booker SE, Israni AK, Hirose R, Snyder JJ. OPTN/SRTR 2019 annual data report. Kidney. 2021;21:21–137.

3. Formica RN Jr, Barrantes F, Asch WS, Bia MJ, Coca S, Kalyesubula R, McCloskey B, Leary T, Arvelakis A, Kulkarni S. A one-day centralized work-up for kidney transplant recipient candidates: a quality improvement report. Am J Kidney Dis. 2012;60:288–94.
4. Harrison JH, Merrill JP, Murray JE. Renal homotransplantation in identical twins. Surg Forum. 1956;6:432–6.
5. Vincenti F, Rostaing L, Grinyo J, Rice K, Steinberg S, Gaite L, Moal M-C, Mondragon-Ramirez GA, Kothari J, Polinsky MS, Meier-Kriesche H-U, Munier S, Larsen CP. Belatacept and long-term outcomes in kidney transplantation. N Engl J Med. 2016;374:333–43.
6. Salani M, Roy S, Fissell WHIV. Innovations in wearable and implantable artificial kidneys. Am J Kidney Dis. 2018;72:745–51.

Chapter 8
Blood Pressure Measurement in Chronic Kidney Disease and End Stage Renal Disease

Stephanie Cardona and Jason Lazar

Introduction

Hypertension has been considered a well-established risk factor for cardiovascular events and mortality in chronic kidney disease (CKD) as well as in patients with end-stage renal disease (ESRD) on hemodialysis. Concurrently, there is a synergistic association between hypertension and diabetes, illustrating how paramount blood pressure (BP) control is for preventing the progression of diabetic nephropathy - the largest subgroup of CKD patients around the world [1]. According to the KDIGO 2012 guidelines [1], CKD is defined as "abnormalities of kidney structure or function that are present for >3 months, with implication to health." There exist a variety of markers that are commonly used to identify CKD including albuminuria, urine sediment abnormalities, electrolyte abnormalities due to tubular disorders, blood urea and creatinine values, histological abnormalities, structural abnormalities on imaging, and a history of kidney transplantation along with a decrease in GFR to less than 60 ml/min/1.73 m [2]. The use of these differing criteria has complicated the assessment of Bp control in terms of slowing CKD progression is less established. For example, while albuminuria is considered a valid surrogate endpoint for certain types of kidney disease [3], whether maximizing therapy to reduce albuminuria in addition to BP control, especially RAAS blockers, is safe or effective in improving clinical outcomes is still unknown.

Blood pressure management is an important consideration along the continuum of CKD including those with ESRD on hemodialysis as BP elevation is quite common in such patients and portends higher rates of cardiovascular and

S. Cardona · J. Lazar (✉)
Division of Cardiology, State University of New York Downstate Health Sciences University, Brooklyn, NY, USA
e-mail: stephanie.cardona@downstate.edu; jason.lazar@downstate.edu

S. J. Saggi, M. O. Salifu (eds.), *Technological Advances in Care of Patients with Kidney Diseases*, https://doi.org/10.1007/978-3-031-11942-2_8

cerebrovascular risk, as well as more rapid CKD progression. While guidelines (KDIGO) for monitoring and establishing BP baselines in patients with CKD have been published, there is less of a consensus for patients with ESRD on hemodialysis. In this chapter, we will briefly: (1) review current guidelines for the management of blood pressure in both the CKD and ESRD populations; (2) provide an overview of technological advancements in BP monitoring used in the office and ambulatory setting; (3) review previously accepted hypertensive markers (BP load, BP variability, arterial stiffness); and (4) elucidate the changes and progression in thinking regarding models of hypertension. While crucial for the management of CKD and ESRD, discussion and review of different pharmacology options for hypertensive management is extensive and thus, beyond the scope of this chapter.

BP Management (Guidelines and Methods)

The basic management strategy of hypertension in CKD and ESRD patients is similar to non-renal disease patients and aims to promote lifestyle modifications and drug therapy to reduce BP [1]. In 2012, Kidney Disease: Improving Global Outcomes (KDIGO) published clinical practice guidelines on the management of BP in non-dialysis CKD [2]. However, an exact threshold for initiating BP lowering therapy and a target BP level has been difficult to determine [1]. Because hypertensive patients frequently have comorbidities including diabetes, cardiovascular and cerebrovascular disease, ideal BP targets may also vary. Therefore, a general strategy of tailoring BP management according to individual risk has been advocated in CKD patients based upon age, co-existing comorbidities (diabetes), risk of progression to CKD, and tolerance of treatment [1]. The management of hypertension in patients with CKD could be viewed to parallel the management of hypertension in the general population. Both higher systolic BP and diastolic BP has been found associated with increasing ESRD risk [4]. Also, while CKD patients comprise a high-risk population resulting in more stringent BP targets advocated for such patients, this recommendation has been called into question as the risk of progression to ESRD was found to start at a systolic BP of 140 mm [4]. Measurement and management of hypertension has been more difficult to define in the ESRD population. In the ESRD population on dialysis, there are frequent and dramatic fluctuations of BP that occur throughout the dialysis cycle. In patients treated with hemodialysis typically 3 days a week, BP progressively rises between sessions because of intravascular volume accumulation and subsequently decreases just after sessions. Additionally, in the hemodialysis population the relationship between BP and outcomes is less straightforward as there appears to be U-shaped relationship between BP and mortality risk with a wide range of nadir risk, which is likely related to the presence of cardiovascular comorbidities in patients with the lowest BPs [5]. In fact, the value of office BP measurement has been called into question as BP elevation in hemodialysis patients is associated with cardiovascular events and mortality when BP is recorded by home measurement or ambulatory monitoring, but not when determined in the dialysis unit [6]. These data infer that pre- and post-dialysis measurements might not reliably reflect BP levels during the interdialytic interval [7]. In this regard, median intradialytic systolic BP has been proposed as a valid estimate of inter-dialytic BP levels compared with peri-dialytic BP measurements. Therefore, median intradialytic SBP can provide a better estimate of interdialytic BP levels compared with peri-dialytic BP measurements [8]. KDOQI guidelines (2015) acknowledge that hypertension affects 60–90% of hemodialysis patients but asserts that the clinical benefits of treating hypertension in patients undergoing hemodialysis have not been established [9]. Furthermore, specific targets for patients on dialysis are not recommended as the BP target that improves hemodialysis outcomes is unknown [10]. Observational studies consistently show poorer survival with pre-dialysis BP <140/90 mmHg, although such studies likely are confounded by low BP due to cardiovascular disease and other comorbidities [7]. Clearly, multiple questions remain about mitigating the risk of BP elevation in this patient population that are perhaps the most vulnerable to further target organ disease resulting from hypertension.

Regarding office-based BP determinations, there are three types of measurement: routine or casual, standardized or the manual technique, and automated oscillometric with a 5-min rest followed by an average of two to three recordings. Casual office BP is generally 5–10 mmHg higher than both standardized office and automated oscillometric office measurements. However, standardized office blood pressure measurements are typically similar to those of automated oscillometric office measurements. In patients with CKD, out-of-office blood pressure may better predict kidney disease progression and cardiovascular events than office measurements. Specifically, ambulatory BP monitoring remains the gold standard to quantify BP load applied to the cardiovascular system [11]. Ambulatory BP monitoring (over 24 h) and self-recorded measurements (over days to weeks) offer the advantage of multiple BP recordings over a single BP measurement is measured in the office setting. From multiple recordings, additional parameters may be derived to portend incremental predictive value above BP level alone.

Blood Pressure Load

Blood pressure load is a parameter that was previously popularized in the early 2000s. It is calculated as the percentage of BP values exceeding a certain threshold over a 24-hour period and is sometimes provided on a report of ambulatory BP monitoring [12]. The BP load accounts for variability in BP values and was proposed to reflect the proportion of time that BP values are abnormally elevated. Several studies have found this parameter predictive of abnormal left ventricular structure and function in hypertensive patients [12, 13]. Accepted thresholds include BP values exceeding 140/90 mmHg while awake and greater than 120/80 mmHg during sleeping hours, or the integrated area under the BP curve above the same cut-offs [12]. While higher BP load has been found to be predictive of the presence and progression of CKD, there is little data as to the value of BP load value in the setting of ESRD.

Blood Pressure Variability

Blood pressure can vary in the short term (minute-to-minute), medium term (day-to-day), or long term (visit-to-visit) variability. These variations have been shown to be the result of complex interactions between extrinsic environmental and behavioral factors, and intrinsic cardiovascular regulatory mechanisms [14]. Models of short-term BP variability include white coat hypertension, masked hypertension, nocturnal and morning hypertension. Although ambulatory BP measurement is considered the gold standard for evaluating hypertension, some studies suggest the application of blood pressure variability is of pathophysiological and prognostic importance [15]. For any given BP value, variability in ambulatory monitoring is associated with a risk for higher rates of adverse outcomes. Blood pressure variability is an important risk factor for cardiovascular events and is associated with higher rates of death and hemorrhagic stroke in patients with moderate to advanced chronic kidney disease not yet on dialysis [16]. More advanced CKD is associated with higher visit-to-visit variability of systolic BP, and higher visit-to-visit variability in CKD is associated with adverse cardiovascular outcomes, adverse renal outcomes, and death. Blood pressure visit-to-visit variability has additionally been shown to be extremely high in hemodialysis patients when compared to other groups, and a major determinant of cardiovascular events in this population [17]. These findings mirror those of those studied in other patient populations.

Arterial Stiffness

In recent years, technical innovations such as applanation tonometry have allowed for the measurement of physical properties such as arterial stiffness. Premature vascular aging and arterial stiffening are characteristic features commonly observed in patients within the early stages of CKD. Arterial stiffening refers to resistance to deformation or a loss of elastic compliance due to changes of the geometry and microstructure of the arterial wall [18]. Stiffness manifests as the change in arterial pressure change resulting from ejection of stroke volume, as well as earlier and more pronounced arterial BP wave reflections. Reflected waves then sum on the next incident pressure wave and increase systolic load on the heart. After contraction of the left ventricle, as much as half of stroke volume is stored within the aorta as it distends. This allows for forward blood flow during diastole. Arterial stiffening increases BP and the increment becomes more pronounced in the aorta and larger arteries than in peripheral conduit arteries, which in turn leads to less protection of the microcirculation in the event of high pressure. Aortic stiffening is associated with high characteristic impedance, left ventricular hypertrophy, decreased coronary perfusion, and is a strong prognostic marker of mortality and cardiovascular morbidity [19]. Arterial stiffening is multifactorial with systemic microinflammation being one of the most important associated factors primarily associated with vascular calcification [17]. Applanation tonometry allows for the precise timing of the upstroke of the arterial BP waveform, which allows for the calculation of pulse wave velocity, a direct measure of arterial stiffness. Among CKD patients, arterial stiffening measured by pulse wave velocity is linked to decreased glomerular filtration rate and is predictive of kidney disease progression [20]. Among CKD and ESRD, increased arterial stiffness is in part related to arterial calcifications [20]. Also, as arterial stiffness is age-dependent, age and carotid-to-femoral pulse wave velocity have been found correlated in both ESRD and control patients with a greater rate of rise observed in the ESRD group [19]. Of note, kidney transplantation improves arterial stiffness in patients with end-stage renal disease [21].

HTN Old-School Vs. New-School Thinking

The old school model for blood pressure considers hypertension as being a systemic disease, in which arterial hemodynamics are altered. The goals of treatment are to directly treat the BP with BP lowering drugs including beta-blockers, angiotensin-converting-enzyme (ACE) inhibitors, angiotensin-receptor blockers (ARBs), diuretics, calcium channel blockers, and others. The new school model views hypertension as a disease of the blood vessels, in which alterations to vascular biology lead to increased arterial stiffness, which in turn increases BP and portends target organ disease. In this model, BP is a biomarker that varies more markedly in CKD and ESRD patients. The goal of management in this model of hypertension is therefore to treat the vasculature using the same drugs used to lower BP.

Summary

Hypertension has long been established as a common and robust risk factor for cardiovascular adverse events in patients with CKD and ESRD. In the case of CKD, the KDIGO guidelines are often applied in practice for appropriate management and treatment of hypertension by individualizing BP targets according to age, existing comorbidities, stage of CKD, presence of diabetes mellitus, and overall treatment tolerance. However, in part due to the frequent and dramatic BP fluctuations that occur during the hemodialysis cycle in patients with ESRD, currently no guidelines are available for determining optimal blood pressure targets that improves outcomes in hemodialysis. Ambulatory blood pressure monitoring is considered the gold standard for measuring the BP load applied to the cardiovascular system and providing an accurate diagnosis of hypertension. While the hypertensive model has been redefined as direct injury of the blood vessels that results in remodeling of vascular biology and changes in arterial stiffness, management of hypertension continues to consist of lifestyle modifications and similar pharmacological therapeutics. The mechanisms and management of hypertension in hemodialysis are yet to be fully elucidated but may be related to factors including volume overload and arterial stiffness. Prompt management and maintenance of adequate BP levels are, therefore, paramount in preventing the high cardiovascular risk associated with CKD and ESRD.

References

1. KDIGO. 2012. BP management in CKD patients. https://kdigo.org/wp-content/uploads/2016/10/KDIGO-2012-Blood-Pressure-Guideline-English.pdf.
2. KDIGO. 2012. CKD guidelines. https://kdigo.org/wp-content/uploads/2017/02/KDIGO_2012_CKD_GL.pdf.
3. Heerspink HJ, Kröpelin TF, Hoekman J, de Zeeuw D. Reducing albuminuria as surrogate endpoint (REASSURE) consortium. Drug-induced reduction in albuminuria is associated with subsequent renoprotection: a meta-analysis. J Am Soc Nephrol. 2015;26(8):2055–64.
4. Peralta CA, Norris KC, Li S, Chang TI, Tamura MK, Jolly SE, Bakris G, McCullough PA, Shlipak M, Investigators KEEP. Blood pressure components and end-stage renal disease in persons with chronic kidney disease: the kidney early evaluation program (KEEP). Arch Intern Med. 2012;172(1):41–7. https://doi.org/10.1001/archinternmed.2011.619.
5. Luther JM. Blood pressure targets in hemodialysis patients. Kidney Int. 2008;73:667–8.
6. Parati G. Hypertension in chronic kidney disease, part 1. Hypertension. 2016;67(6):1093–101. https://doi.org/10.1161/HYPERTENSIONAHA.115.06895.
7. Loutradis CN, Tsioufis C, Sarafidis PA. The clinical problems of hypertension treatment in hemodialysis patients. Curr Vasc Pharmacol. 2017;16(1):54–60.
8. Georgianos PI, Agarwal R. Blood pressure in hemodialysis: targets? Curr Opin Nephrol Hypertens. 2017;26(6):523–9. https://doi.org/10.1097/MNH.0000000000000359.
9. KDOQI. 2015 guideline for HD adequacy. https://www.ajkd.org/action/showPdf?pii=S02726386%2815%2901019-7.
10. Miskulin DC, Weiner DE. Blood pressure management in hemodialysis patients: what we know and what questions remain. Semin Dial. 2017;30(3):203–12.
11. Saint-Remy A, Krzesinski JM. Optimal blood pressure level and best measurement procedure in hemodialysis patients. Vasc Health Risk Manag. 2005;1(3):235–44.
12. Liu M, Li Y, Wei FF, Zhang L, Han JL, Wang JG. Is blood pressure load associated, independently of blood pressure level, with target organ damage? J Hypertens. 2013;31(9):1812–8.
13. White WB. Blood pressure load and target organ effects in patients with essential hypertension. J Hypertens Suppl. 1991;9(8):S39–41.
14. Parati G, Ochoa JE, Lombardi C, Bilo G. Assessment and management of blood-pressure variability [published correction appears in Nat Rev Cardiol. 2014;11(6):314]. Nat Rev Cardiol. 2013;10(3):143–55.
15. Chadachan VM, Ye MT, Tay JC, Subramaniam K, Setia S. Understanding short-term blood-pressure-variability phenotypes: from concept to clinical practice. Int J Gen Med. 2018;11:241–54.

16. Chang TI, Tabada GH, Yang J, Tan TC, Go AS. Visit-to-visit variability of blood pressure and death, end-stage renal disease, and cardiovascular events in patients with chronic kidney disease. J Hypertens. 2016;34(2):244–52.
17. Rossignol P, Cridlig J, Lehert P, Kessler M, Zannad F. Visit-to-visit blood pressure variability is a strong predictor of cardiovascular events in hemodialysis: insights from FOSIDIAL. Hypertension. 2012;60(2):339–46.
18. Ogola BO, Zimmerman MA, Clark GL, et al. New insights into arterial stiffening: does sex matter? Am J Physiol Heart Circ Physiol. 2018;315(5):H1073–87.
19. London GM. Arterial stiffness in chronic kidney disease and end-stage renal disease. Blood Purif. 2018;45(1–3):154–8.
20. Briet M, Boutouyrie P, Laurent S, London GM. Arterial stiffness and pulse pressure in CKD and ESRD. Kidney Int. 2012;82(4):388–400. https://doi.org/10.1038/ki.2012.131.
21. Feng S, Wang H, Yang J, Hu X, Wang W, Liu H, Li H, Zhang X. Kidney transplantation improves arterial stiffness in patients with end-stage renal disease. Int Urol Nephrol. 2020;52(5):877–84. https://doi.org/10.1007/s11255-020-02376-3.

Chapter 9
Assessing Volume Overload in Patients on Dialysis

Akbar Hamid and Tariq Shafi

Introduction

Patients with end stage kidney disease (ESKD) have high health burden—including comorbidities and complex medication regimes. Hospitalizations and emergency visits are also common in patients on dialysis and volume overload is a major contributor. The exact burden of volume overload is difficult to quantify, but if we take incident heart failure in patients with ESKD as a proxy for volume overload, about 50% of patients on hemodialysis and 36% of patients on peritoneal dialysis are diagnosed with heart failure within 2 years of starting dialysis (Fig. 9.1).

The two goals of dialysis treatments are to remove uremic toxins and achieve euvolemia. The latter goal has been difficult to achieve due to several factors including our inability to reliably assess volume in patients on dialysis. Volume overload in patients on dialysis results in persistent hypertension, left ventricular hypertrophy, heart failure, and arrhythmias. However, rapid fluid removal during dialysis treatment can cause complications including intradialytic hypotension, myocardial stunning, stroke, dialysis access thrombosis, and faster decline in residual kidney function (Fig. 9.2). Volume assessment precedes every single dialysis treatment but our clinical methods for assessing volume are limited to detecting florid volume

A. Hamid
Division of Nephrology, Department of Medicine, SUNY Downstate Health Sciences University, Brooklyn, NY, USA
e-mail: Akbar.Hamid@downstate.edu

T. Shafi (✉)
Division of Nephrology, Department of Medicine, University of Mississippi Medical Center, Jackson, MS, USA
e-mail: tshafi@umc.edu

S. J. Saggi, M. O. Salifu (eds.), *Technological Advances in Care of Patients with Kidney Diseases*, https://doi.org/10.1007/978-3-031-11942-2_9

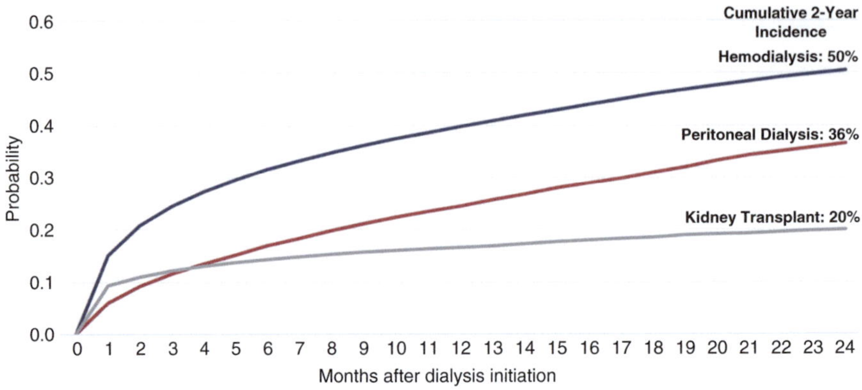

Fig. 9.1 Unadjusted 2-year incidence of heart failure in patients with ESRD, 2016–2018. Adapted from the 2020 United States Renal Data System Annual Data Report, Fig. 8.6

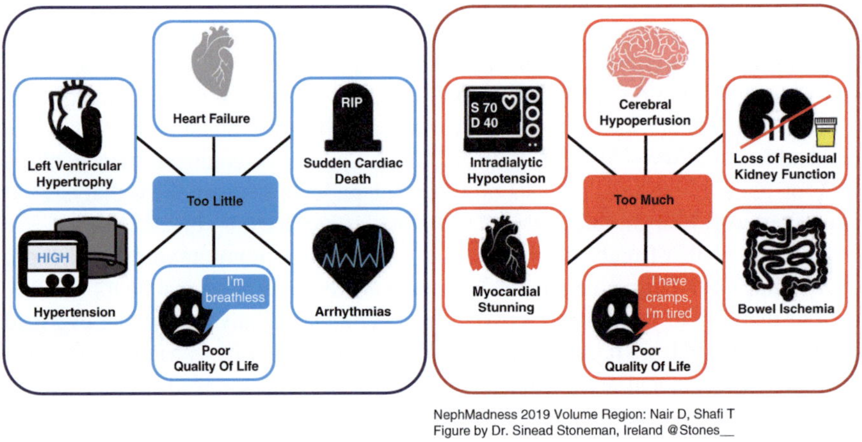

Fig. 9.2 The volume management conundrum in patients on dialysis. The figure illustrates the potential risks associated with either suboptimal volume removal or excessive volume removal. Source: Figure created by Dr. Sinead Stoneman for NephMadness 2019 (https://ajkdblog.org/2019/03/15/nephmadness-2019-volume-assessment-region/)

overload. In this review, we will briefly review the physiology of volume overload and discuss new techniques to objectively assess volume which could be applied to caring for patients on dialysis.

Physiology

In healthy individuals, total body water accounts for about 60% of the body weight; 40% in the intracellular compartment and 20% in the extracellular compartment (Fig. 9.3). The extracellular fluid volume (ECFV) expands to accommodate volume

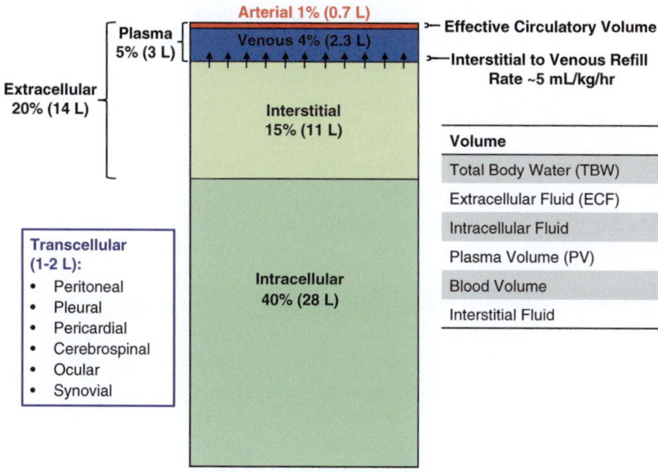

Volume	Measurement Method
Total Body Water (TBW)	$^{3}H_2O$, Ethanol
Extracellular Fluid (ECF)	Iohexol, inulin
Intracellular Fluid	=TBW-ECF
Plasma Volume (PV)	^{125}I Albumin, Evans blue
Blood Volume	=PV/(1-hematocrit)
Interstitial Fluid	=ECF-PV

Fig. 9.3 Body fluid compartments and distribution of water in a 70 kg person. Table describes methods for measuring each of the fluid compartment

overload in disease states. Of the ECFV, only 5% or 3 L is the plasma volume with just 700 mL in the arterial circuit and the remaining 2.3 L in the venous circuit. Ultrafiltration during hemodialysis often exceeds 700 mL/min and maintaining plasma volume and blood pressure during this rapid removal is driven by several factors. If the fluid removal rate on dialysis exceeds the interstitial to venous refill rate, hypotension occurs, its timing determined further by interstitial to venous compartment refill, vascular compliance, cardiac function, and integrity of the autonomic nervous system [1].

Devices to Assess Volume

In routine clinical practice, the presence and severity of volume overload in patients on dialysis is assessed by a combination of physical examination findings, such as edema, dyspnea, and hypertension, combined with the increase in weight between dialysis treatments. A number of existing and emerging technologies are available that can allow further refinement of volume assessment (Table 9.1).

Bioimpedance

Bioimpedance is noninvasive, safe, easy, portable, and relatively inexpensive. It requires placement of electrodes on the body and measures tissue conductivity in response to a small bioelectrical current. Tissue conductivity is directly proportional to the amount of electrolyte-containing fluid present and the frequency of electrical

Table 9.1 Volume assessment methods and their advantages and limitations

Volume assessment method	Body fluid compartment assessed	Advantages	Limitations
Weight, BP, edema, crackles	Total body water Interstitial fluid	Simplicity, sufficient for florid volume overload	Inability to distinguish between subtle changes
Whole body bioimpedance	Total body water Intracellular fluid	Simple, non-invasive	Lack of validity: Diverse populations, ESKD, subtle changes
Thoracic electrical bioimpedance	Lung interstitial fluid	Simple, non-invasive	Other fluid compartments are not assessed; validity in ESKD is not known
Remote dielectric sensing	Lung interstitial fluid	Simple, non-invasive, does not require electric current	Other fluid compartments are not assessed; validity in ESKD is not known
Blood volume monitoring	Blood volume, interstitial to venous refill	Non-invasive (used with dialysis circuit); data available in real-time	Interpretation and ultrafiltration modification requires training
Point of care ultrasound	Venous compartment (inferior vena cava) and lung interstitial fluid	Non-invasive, portable devices	Image acquisition and interpretation requires extensive training
CardioMEMS	Pulmonary artery pressure (venous compartment)	Real-time monitoring of pulmonary artery pressure	Invasive procedure to implant device (right heart catheterization)

Abbreviations: *BP* blood pressure, *ESKD* end-stage kidney disease

current. Low frequency current allows estimation of the extracellular water, high frequency current allows estimation of total body water and the intracellular water is calculated by subtracting the two values. The equations for calculating (estimating) the fluid compartments are derived from healthy people and their validity in patients on dialysis is not well-described. Accuracy of bioimpedance during the dynamic fluid compartment changes during hemodialysis is also not known [2, 3].

Thoracic Electrical Bioimpedance

Thoracic electrical bioimpedance was first developed in the 1960s to enable remote non-invasive monitoring the cardiac status of astronauts. Like the whole body bioimpedance, focused thoracic bioimpedance could provide information on congestion. Several thoracic bioimpedance devices have been tested and trials of the efficacy of this technique to guide fluid management in heart failure, are ongoing [4, 5].

Blood Volume Monitoring

In contrast to bioimpedance, blood volume monitoring is designed to estimate the volume of the intravascular compartment. Absolute blood volume monitoring uses the indicator dilution technique, using ultrapure dialysate, to calculate each patient's blood volume. The more frequently used relative blood monitoring non-invasively assesses the hemoconcentration of the blood in the dialysis circuit to estimate the blood volume. Three relative blood volume monitoring device are available. The Crit-Line monitor uses an optical sensor to detect changes in hematocrit. The Hemoscan uses the optical absorbance of hemoglobin to estimate blood volume and the Fresenius Blood Volume Monitor uses ultrasonic technology to estimate the concentration of proteins and hemoglobin, inferring blood volume. Realtime monitoring of the blood volume (in the dialysis circuit) can identify patients with rapid reduction of blood volume and potentially prevent intradialytic hypotension by reducing ultrafiltration. However, the clinical studies of the effectiveness are equivocal [6, 7].

Ultrasound

Point-of-care ultrasound (POCUS) is now widely available. POCUS assessment of volume includes counting B-lines and measuring the inferior vena cava (IVC). The B-lines are sonographic manifestation of thickened interlobular septa or fluid-filled alveoli. Rigorous assessment of B-lines requires counting the number of lines at 28 sites in eight regions of the chest, but is rarely done in routine clinical practice. The IVC diameter > 2.5 cm, without inspiratory collapse, suggests venous congestion which could be from volume overload. A large ongoing European trial is assessing the feasibility and efficacy of lung ultrasound assessment in managing volume in patients on dialysis and should provide more insights into the use of lung ultrasound in outpatient hemodialysis settings [8].

CardioMEMS

CardioMEMS is a device implanted in the pulmonary artery during right heart catheterization and provides data similar to a Swan Ganz catheter. Changes in pulmonary artery pressure, indicating changes in volume and congestion, can be non-invasively monitored by the patient. CardioMEMS is widely used for management of patients with heart failure and has potential to guide fluid management in patients on dialysis [9, 10].

Remote Dielectric Sensing (ReDS)

ReDS technology measures the dielectric properties of tissues. Low-power electromagnetic signals are sent through the lungs using two sensors that can be placed on top of clothing. The characteristics of the signals received after passing through the tissues are related to their dielectric properties which, in turn, are mostly determined by the lung's fluid content. ReDS quantifies lung congestion at the right middle lobe of the lung. The device is undergoing efficacy studies in patients with heart failure [11].

Indicor (Investigational Use)

The Indicor is a noninvasive device that assesses changes in pulse amplitude ratio in response to a Valsalva maneuver. The pulse amplitude ratio is a non-invasive method to gauge the left ventricular end-diastolic pressure, reflecting left ventricular filling pressures and volume overload. The device is undergoing efficacy testing in heart failure. Preliminary findings in patients on dialysis were equivocal [12].

Conclusion

Volume overload is a major challenge to the appropriate management of patients on dialysis. Objective methods to assess volume status and achieve euvolemia are critical to improving care of patients on dialysis. The emerging methods and devices to assess volume status require former testing and efficacy studies in patients on dialysis. It is time to step up and move beyond the sole emphasis on the weighing scale and the ultrafiltration rate as the only methods to manage volume overload.

References

1. Hall JE. Guyton and Hall textbook of medical physiology. 13th ed. 2015: Saunders; 1168.
2. Moissl UM, et al. Body fluid volume determination via body composition spectroscopy in health and disease. Physiol Meas. 2006;27(9):921–33.
3. Earthman C, et al. Bioimpedance spectroscopy for clinical assessment of fluid distribution and body cell mass. Nutr Clin Pract. 2007;22(4):389–405.
4. Broomhead CJ, et al. Thoracic electrical bioimpedance: a non-invasive measure of cardiac output for porcine research. Lab Anim. 1998;32(3):324–9.
5. Shochat MK, et al. Non-invasive lung IMPEDANCE-guided preemptive treatment in chronic heart failure patients: a randomized controlled trial (IMPEDANCE-HF trial). J Card Fail. 2016;22(9):713–22.

6. Crit-Line® III monitor frequently asked questions. 2015. https://fmcna.com/content/dam/fmcna/live/support/documents/fluid-management/crit-line-iii/Crit-Line%20III%20FAQs.pdf.
7. Balter P, Artemyev M, Zabetakis P. Methods and challenges for the practical application of Crit-line™ monitor utilization in patients on hemodialysis. Blood Purif. 2015;39(1–3):21–4.
8. Loutradis C, et al. The effect of dry-weight reduction guided by lung ultrasound on ambulatory blood pressure in hemodialysis patients: a randomized controlled trial. Kidney Int. 2019;95(6):1505–13.
9. Yevzlin AS, Valliant AM. Interventional nephrology: novel devices that will one day change our practice. Clin J Am Soc Nephrol. 2013;8(7):1244–51.
10. Abraham WT, et al. Wireless pulmonary artery haemodynamic monitoring in chronic heart failure: a randomised controlled trial. Lancet. 2011;377(9766):658–66.
11. Amir O, et al. A novel approach to monitoring pulmonary congestion in heart failure: initial animal and clinical experiences using remote dielectric sensing technology. Congest Heart Fail. 2013;19(3):149–55.
12. Galiatsatos P, et al. A finger photoplethysmography waveform during the valsalva maneuver detects changes in left heart filling pressure after hemodialysis. BMC Nephrol. 2015;16:138.

Chapter 10
Technologies to Monitor Dialysis Dose, Vascular Access Function and Improve Toxin Removal

Shakil Aslam, Subodh J. Saggi, and Moro O. Salifu

Introduction

Blood urea-based measurements are the most commonly used and clinically validated methods to monitor dialysis adequacy, although urea is just one of several potential uremic toxins. Urea is a good surrogate of small, water-soluble compounds; however, larger molecules such as β2-microglobulin and protein-bound uremic toxins likely contribute to morbidity and mortality in patients with ESKD. Kt/V_{Urea} is the preferred method of quantifying the dose of delivered dialysis. A single pool Kt/V ($spKt/V_{urea}$) of 1.2 is considered the minimally adequate and recommended dose of hemodialysis per session for patients receiving thrice-weekly dialysis [1]. A target $spKt/V_{Urea}$ of 1.4 should be prescribed to achieve the target of 1.2. Typically blood urea-based Kt/V measurements are performed only once or twice monthly with no way of ensuring that the dialysis adequacy target was met for all dialysis treatments. Furthermore, the results cannot be used to modify an ongoing dialysis treatment. Most modern hemodialysis machines incorporate technologies to estimate Kt/V online during a dialysis session. Currently, there are no methods available for routine clinical use to measure the dialytic removal of middle molecules and protein-bound toxins. Due to differences in dialyzability, different strategies are needed to optimize the removal of urea, middle molecules, and protein-bound toxins.

S. Aslam (✉)
Angion Biomedica Corp, Uniondale, NY, USA
e-mail: saslam@angion.com

S. J. Saggi · M. O. Salifu
Medicine, SUNY Downstate Health Sciences University, Brooklyn, NY, USA

Medicine, SUNY Downstate Medical Center, Brooklyn, NY, USA
e-mail: subodh.saggi@downstate.edu; moro.salifu@downstate.edu

S. J. Saggi, M. O. Salifu (eds.), *Technological Advances in Care of Patients with Kidney Diseases*, https://doi.org/10.1007/978-3-031-11942-2_10

Technologies for Online Monitoring of Dialysis Dose

Currently, two technologies are available for estimating the dialysis dose "online" in real time; the effective ionic dialysance (EID) of Na^+-based methods such as Diascan™ (Baxter, Deerfield, IL, USA) and Online Clearance Monitoring (OCM™) and Online Clearance (OLC™) (Fresenius Medical Care, Waltham, MA, USA), and ultraviolet (UV) spectrophotometry-based systems such as Adimea™ (B. Braun, Hessen, Germany) and Dialysis Dose Monitor™ (Nikkiso, Tokyo, Japan), which measure the absorbance of the spent dialysate. The principles and operating characteristics of these technologies are summarized in Table 10.1.

EID-Na^+ Based Methods

This method measures the dialysance of Na^+ to estimate urea clearance. Sodium ions and urea exhibit comparable diffusion characteristics across a dialyzer membrane. Their specific diffusion coefficient is almost identical at 37 °C.

Table 10.1 Comparison of two currently used technologies for on-line dialysis adequacy monitoring

	UV spectrophotometric method	Ionic or Na^+ dialysance
Principle	UV spectrophotometric monitoring of spent dialysate for the removal of "uremic toxins"	Determination of dialyzer Na^+ conductance as a measure of urea clearance
Operating characteristics and key features	Continuously measures the spent dialysate's absorbance to calculate Kt/V and URR	Measures dialyzer's clearance (K) intermittently at the given Qb and Qd to calculate Kt/V
	Volume of distribution (V) does not need to be entered	Requires the user to enter patient's "V" to calculate Kt/V, prone to errors
	Provides an estimate of the delivered dose, adjusts for changes in K	Provides a theoretical Kt/V based on the dialyzer clearance at pre-programmed intervals
	The UV wavelength used is not specific for urea	Does not measure urea clearance. Uses Na^+/ionic dialysance as a surrogate for urea clearance
	Cannot be used for estimating the dialysis access blood flow rate	Can be used to measure dialysis access blood flow rate with certain limitations
	A deterioration in the dialyzer performance not easy to detect and can overestimate the delivered dose of dialysis	A deterioration in the dialyzer performance easy to detect by a drop in Na^+ dialysance

During a measurement, the dialysate conductivity, which is mostly represented by its Na^+ concentration, is transiently increased to 15.5 mS/cm. This approximates a dialysate Na^+ concentration of 155 mEq/L. The dialysate Na^+ moves across the dialyzer membrane into the blood resulting in a drop in the spent dialysate conductivity, which is detected by an additional conductivity sensor in the spent dialysate path. In some machines, in a second step, the dialysate conductivity is transiently lowered to 13.5 mS/cm allowing the movement of Na^+ in the opposite direction from blood to the dialysate, which increases the spent dialysate conductivity. The change in dialysate conductivity is used to calculate the "conductivity clearance, $K_{ecn,}$" which is considered equivalent to the urea clearance (K_{urea}). The programmed duration of the dialysis treatment provides "t" to calculate the K_{ecn}t. The volume "V" is manually entered into the machine to calculate the K_{ecn}t/V.

The Kt/V value derived from EID-based methods generally correlates well with the Kt/V_{urea} [2]; however, certain limitations must be recognized. The volume "V" entered manually can introduce significant error or variability. Anthropometric formulas such as Watson's formula overestimate "V" in dialysis patients and their use can underestimate the delivered K_{ecn}t/V compared to spKt/V_{urea} [3]. The second generation Daugirdas equation for Kt/V may be more accurate and easier to use to calculate "V". EID does not measure the delivered dialysis dose; it merely measures the performance of the dialyzer at given blood and dialysate flow rates at preprogrammed intervals (typically every 30 minutes) and projects the delivered dose. The initially projected dose may not be delivered if the clearance decreases due to clotting of the dialyzer or if the same blood or dialysate flow rates are not maintained between measurements. Since measurements are made only intermittently, the effects of an intervention on the clearance cannot be seen until the next measurement.

EID can also be used to measure the access flow, although the precision decreases when the access flow rate exceeds 1000 mL/min [4].

There have been some concerns about the potential of salt loading with EID-based methods; however, there appears to be no evidence of a clinically meaningful salt loading during these measurements [5, 6].

UV Spectrophotometry-based Method

This method utilizes UV-spectrophotometry for determining the reduction in the molar concentration of several small molecules in the spent dialysate during a dialysis session. Although the UV wavelength used is not specific for urea, a good correlation (0.93) has been reported between blood urea-based Kt/V and UV-spectrophotometry-based Kt/V [7]. This method offers some advantages over the EID-based methods. No entry of volume (V) is required; only pre-dialysis weight needs to be entered. This method provides a measurement of the delivered dose, which can be expressed as urea reduction ratio or spKt/V. This method can be used to estimate the protein catabolic rate. Since monitoring occurs continuously, the effects of any changes to the flow rates on the clearance can be assessed in real-time.

The UV-spectrophotometry-based method cannot be used to monitor the access blood flow rate.

Optimizing Dialysis Dose

The delivered Kt/V_{urea} can be increased by increasing the clearance (K) and/or the duration of the dialysis session (t). The clearance (K) can be increased by increasing the blood flow rate (Qb), the dialysate flow rate (Qd), or by using a larger dialyzer. However, there are limitations to the degree of improvement these measures can achieve. Improvements in the clearance are rather modest beyond the Qb of 400 mL/min, Qd of 600 mL/min or the dialyzer surface area beyond 2.0 m^2. There may also be unintended consequences of increasing Qb to optimize clearance. High Qb can increase access recirculation in vascular accesses with a restricted blood flow and increase the generation of microbubbles, which are below the detection limit of the air-bubble detectors [8]. Larger dialyzers require higher doses of anticoagulants, and an uneven blood and dialysate flow distribution may reduce their efficiency.

Many modern hemodialysis machines offer "autoflow" function, where the dialysate flow rate can be automatically adjusted as a multiple of the Qb. The dialysate flow rate greater than 1.5 × Qb offers only minimal improvement in the clearance and increases dialysate waste [9]. The most efficient and predictable intervention to improve the delivered Kt/V_{urea} is to increase "t," the length of the dialysis session (Table 10.2).

Table 10.2 Various strategies to optimize hemodialysis adequacy

Intervention	Pros	Cons
Use a larger dialyzer	May work if increasing the time on dialysis (t) not possible	Dialyzers become less efficient as the size increases. Very little improvement beyond 2.0 m^2 surface area High Qb and Qd needed to optimize the membrane use and clearance Higher doses of heparin needed Higher cost of the dialyzer
Increase the blood flow rate (Qb)	Optimizes the dialyzer membrane utilization May obviate the need to increase the time on dialysis (t) in some cases	Larger access needles required Clearance does not increase linearly with Qb especially at higher Qb. Very little improvement beyond 400–450 mL/min of Qb Does not improve the clearance of middle molecules or phosphate Recirculation may increase Increased microbubble formation and air infusion

Table 10.2 (continued)

Intervention	Pros	Cons
Increase the dialysate flow rate (Qd)	Optimizes the dialyzer membrane utilization	Not much improvement in clearance at Qd beyond 1.5 × Qb
Increase the duration of dialysis (t)	Best option in large patients Increases the middle molecule and phosphate clearance Ultrafiltration better tolerated Lesser severity of disequilibrium post-dialysis Generally, the simplest and most efficient intervention to improve dialysis adequacy	Poor patient compliance Dialysis unit logistics and cost

Optimizing the Removal of Middle Molecules and Protein-Bound Toxins

The failure to improve clinical outcomes with the delivered Kt/V_{urea} of greater than 1.2 [9] has generated a lot of interest in enhancing the removal of the middle molecules and the protein-bound toxins to improve clinical outcomes. Middle molecules (500 Da to 60 kDa) include several cytokines, adipokines, growth factors, and other signaling proteins that are significantly elevated in patients with ESKD and are implicated in inflammation and atherosclerosis. β2-microglobulin is the most commonly studied middle molecule. Some of the currently available technologies to increase middle molecular clearance are discussed as follows.

High-Flux Dialyzers

High-flux dialyzers have an aqueous ultrafiltration coefficient (K_{uf}) greater than 20 mL/h/mmHg of transmembrane pressure and β2-microglobulin clearance greater than 20 mL/min. These dialyzers provide high convective clearance due to backfiltration or internal filtration. Although the HEMO trial [1] did not show a survival benefit of using high-flux dialyzers, there appeared to be an overall and cardiovascular survival benefit in patients who had been on HD for more than 3.7 years prior to randomization to high-flux dialyzers. However, this interaction was weakened when years on dialysis prior to randomization were treated as a continuous variable or were further subdivided into quintiles. In addition, there was no evidence of a risk reduction for high-flux dialysis, compared with low-flux dialysis, with additional years of dialysis after randomization [10].

On-Line Hemodiafiltration

Online hemodiafiltration (OL-HDF) combines diffusive clearance with large volumes of convective clearance using the replacement fluid generated by the dialysis machines "online." The post-dilution mode of OL-HDF provides the highest clearance of middle molecules, which far exceeds the clearance achieved by high-flux dialyzers alone. Large randomized trials have shown conflicting results on the beneficial effects of OL-HDF on clinical outcomes [11, 12]. Most randomized controlled trials demonstrated an improvement in clinical outcomes only on post-hoc analyses, especially when the convective volume was greater than 23 L/session. The only large randomized controlled trial [12] that showed an improvement in the primary endpoints of all-cause and cardiovascular mortality used a flawed randomization scheme where patients unable to tolerate a trial of hemodiafiltration during the pre-randomization period were assigned to receive hemodialysis. Thus, patients who exhibited hemodynamic instability during a trial of high-volume hemodiafiltration were randomized to receive intermittent hemodialysis, thus introducing a bias in favor of hemodiafiltration.

Post-dilution OL-HDF is associated with marked hemoconcentration in the dialyzer, very high backfiltration, and increased risk of dialyzer clotting and albumin loss. Sophisticated dialyzer pressure monitoring technologies and software algorithms are needed to control filtration fraction to avoid these complications.

Medium Molecular Cut-off Membranes

More recently, dialysis membranes with increased pore size and permeability are being used to achieve middle molecule clearance similar to or better than OL-HDF [13, 14]. Medium cut-off (MCO) membranes can remove molecules >25 kDa in size. MCO membranes have demonstrated greater clearances of α1-microglobulin, complement factor D, kappa FLC (κFLC), and myoglobin than high-flux HD and similar to or greater than clearances with OL-HDF. The use of these membranes can result in a much greater loss of albumin (3–10 g/session) than with high-flux HD and OL-HDF (<1 g/session) [14]. Currently, there is no evidence that using MCO membranes improves clinical outcomes despite higher elimination of middle molecules and larger proteins.

Removal of Protein-Bound Toxins

Protein-bound toxins are poorly removed by any form of dialysis. These toxins range from small uncharged solutes to large protein-bound molecules. Some of the protein-bound uremic toxins, such as indoxyl sulfate and p-cresyl sulfate, have been linked to vascular inflammation, endothelial dysfunction, and vascular calcification [15]. Currently, no technologies exist to remove protein-bound uremic toxins for clinical use. Infusion of "displacers" such as ibuprofen into the arterial bloodline has been shown to improve the clearance of indoxyl sulfate and p-cresyl sulfate [16]. This approach has considerable practical limitations, including the safety of the pharmaceutical displacers and their impact on the protein-bound drugs before the impact of this approach on clinical outcomes could be investigated.

Another approach to increase the dialytic removal of protein-bound toxins is to permit some albumin loss during dialysis using high permeability MCO membranes. The dialytic loss of albumin is hypothesized to result in the loss of protein-bound toxins. The safety, efficiency, and benefits of this approach to remove protein-bound toxins are unproven [17] and warrant further investigation.

In summary, the concentrations of several pro-inflammatory cytokines, middle molecules, and larger proteins are elevated in patients with ESKD and correlate with adverse clinical outcomes. However, the approaches to increase the dialytic removal of these presumed uremic toxins using high-flux dialyzers, OL-HDF, and high permeability membranes have not been shown to improve clinical outcomes in randomized controlled trials. This may be due to the lack of long-term follow-up in these studies. Although some of the newer approaches are very effective in increasing the dialytic elimination of the middle molecules, their effect on the time-averaged concentration of these toxins may be less pronounced due to a significant rebound in their plasma concentrations after a dialysis treatment [18]. Longer and more frequent dialysis treatments are likely to reduce the time-averaged concentration of the middle molecules more effectively.

Despite its limitations, urea kinetic modeling is the most extensively studied and validated method of monitoring dialysis adequacy. Urea clearance cannot be measured directly during a dialysis session; however, safe, reliable, and easy-to-use technologies exist on most modern dialysis machines to monitor dialysis adequacy during a dialysis session. These technologies should be used to complement the dialysis adequacy monitoring based on the urea kinetic modeling to deliver optimal dialysis dose.

References

1. Eknoyan G, Beck GJ, Cheung AK, et al. Effect of dialysis dose and membrane flux in maintenance hemodialysis. N Engl J Med. 2002;347(25):2010–9. https://doi.org/10.1056/NEJMoa021583.
2. Lindsay RM, Bene B, Goux N, Heidenheim AP, Landgren C, Sternby J. Relationship between effective ionic dialysance and in vivo urea clearance during hemodialysis. Am J Kidney Dis. 2001;38(3):565–74. https://doi.org/10.1053/ajkd.2001.26874.
3. Casino FG, Mancini E, Santarsia G, et al. What volume to choose to assess online Kt/V? J Nephrol. 2020;33(1):137–46. https://doi.org/10.1007/s40620-019-00636-9.

4. Lacson E, Lazarus JM, Panlilio R, Gotch F. Comparison of hemodialysis blood access flow rates using online measurement of conductivity dialysance and ultrasound dilution. Am J Kidney Dis. 2008;51(1):99–106. https://doi.org/10.1053/j.ajkd.2007.10.001.
5. Gotch FA, Panlilio FM, Buyaki RA, Wang EX, Folden TI, Levin NW. Mechanisms determining the ratio of conductivity clearance to urea clearance. Kidney Int Suppl. 2004;89:S3–S24.
6. Moret K, Grootendorst DC, Beerenhout C, Kooman JP. Conductivity pulses needed for Diascan measurements: does it cause sodium burden. Clin Kidney J. 2009;2(4):334–5. https://doi.org/10.1093/ndtplus/sfp059.
7. Alex C, Michael W, Roman G, Marten J. Real-time Kt/V determination by ultraviolet absorbance in spent dialysate: technique validation. Kidney Int. 2010;78(9):920–5. https://doi.org/10.1038/ki.2010.216.
8. Stegmayr B, Brännström T, Forsberg U, Jonson P, Stegmayr C, Hultdin J. Microbubbles of air may occur in the organs of hemodialysis patients. ASAIO J. 2012;58(2):177–9. https://doi.org/10.1097/MAT.0b013e318245d0dd.
9. Albalate M, Pérez-García R, de Sequera P, et al. Is it useful to increase dialysate flow rate to improve the delivered Kt? BMC Nephrol. 2015;16:20. https://doi.org/10.1186/s12882-015-0013-9.
10. Cheung AK, Levin NW, Greene T, et al. Effects of high-flux hemodialysis on clinical outcomes: results of the HEMO study. J Am Soc Nephrol. 2003;14(12):3251–63. https://doi.org/10.1097/01.ASN.0000096373.13406.94.
11. Grooteman MPC, van den Dorpel MA, Bots ML, et al. Effect of online hemodiafiltration on all-cause mortality and cardiovascular outcomes. J Am Soc Nephrol. 2012;23(6):1087–96. https://doi.org/10.1681/ASN.2011121140.
12. Maduell F, Moreso F, Pons M, et al. High-efficiency postdilution online hemodiafiltration reduces all-cause mortality in hemodialysis patients. J Am Soc Nephrol. 2013;24(3):487–97. https://doi.org/10.1681/ASN.2012080875.
13. Weiner DE, Falzon L, Skoufos L, et al. Efficacy and safety of expanded hemodialysis with the Theranova 400 dialyzer: a randomized controlled trial. Clin J Am Soc Nephrol. 2020;15(9):1310–9. https://doi.org/10.2215/CJN.01210120.
14. Kirsch AH, Lyko R, Nilsson L-G, et al. Performance of hemodialysis with novel medium cut-off dialyzers. Nephrol Dial Transplant. 2017;32(1):165–72. https://doi.org/10.1093/ndt/gfw310.
15. Barreto FC, Barreto DV, Liabeuf S, et al. Serum indoxyl sulfate is associated with vascular disease and mortality in chronic kidney disease patients. Clin J Am Soc Nephrol. 2009;4(10):1551–8. https://doi.org/10.2215/CJN.03980609.
16. Madero M, Cano KB, Campos I, et al. Removal of protein-bound uremic toxins during hemodialysis using a binding competitor. Clin J Am Soc Nephrol. 2019;14(3):394–402. https://doi.org/10.2215/CJN.05240418.
17. Ward RA. Protein-leaking membranes for hemodialysis: a new class of membranes in search of an application? J Am Soc Nephrol. 2005;16(8):2421–30. https://doi.org/10.1681/ASN.2005010070.
18. Leypoldt John K, Cheung Alfred K, Deeter R. Barry. Rebound kinetics of ß2-microglobulin after hemodialysis. Kidney Int. 1999;56(4):1571–7. https://doi.org/10.1046/j.1523-1755.1999.00669.x.

Chapter 11
Technologies Transforming AV Fistula Creation: "Endo-AVF or Percutaneous-AVF"

David Fox

History of Hemodialysis Access

For over half a century, the native arterio-venous fistula (avf) has been the gold standard of hemodialysis access. The first avf was described by Brescia, Cimino, Hurwich, and Appel in 1966 [1]. Since then, numerous innovations and variations in surgical technique have been introduced, such as transpositions and fistulas based on the proximal radial and ulnar arteries [2, 3].

While innovative, these techniques are all fundamentally open surgical procedures, which have varying degrees of surgical challenge, morbidity, and patient acceptance. In recent years, a new set of concepts and technologies has emerged. These allow the creation of an arteriovenous anastomosis using percutaneous endovascular devices and techniques, thus obviating the need for open surgery for some patients. Fistulas created in this way are known as endovascular av. fistulas, (endo-AVF) or percutaneous av. fistulas (pavf). These innovative techniques hold the promise of decreased surgical morbidity, increased patient acceptance, and perhaps improved maturation and functional patency [4, 5].

The Endo-AVF Concept

Fundamentally, the endo-AVF concept involves utilizing a percutaneously delivered device to create a connection between a deep artery and a deep vein in the proximal forearm. These connections may be between the proximal ulnar artery and the proximal ulnar vein, the proximal radial artery, and the proximal radial vein, or between the proximal radial artery and perforator vein directly. Blood will then flow from the

D. Fox (✉)
Fox Vein and Vascular, New York, NY, USA

S. J. Saggi, M. O. Salifu (eds.), *Technological Advances in Care of Patients with Kidney Diseases*, https://doi.org/10.1007/978-3-031-11942-2_11

deep veins to the superficial veins via the perforator vein in the proximal forearm. Coil embolization or ligation of draining veins is often required to direct sufficient flow to the superficial system that will serve as the cannulation zone for dialysis. If the outflow vein is too deep to allow for cannulation, staged superficialization of the basilic, cephalic or brachial vein is performed after a period of maturation.

Two Technologies

At present, there are two technologies that have been approved by the FDA for endovascular av. fistula creation. These are the Ellipsys (Avenu, now Medtronic Medical) and WavelinQ (Bard) systems. The Ellipsys Vascular Access System consists of a 6 French Thermal Resistance Anastomosis Device (T-RAD) and a power controller. The Ellipsys device creates an immediate and permanent anastomosis between the proximal radial artery and perforator vein via tissue fusion, utilizing pressure and thermal resistance [6]. Angioplasty of the newly formed anastomosis is performed with a 5 mm balloon. Coil embolization of draining veins and superficialization are performed subsequently, on an as-needed basis, to direct flow to the target vein and to facilitate cannulation. The Ellipsys procedure is performed entirely under duplex ultrasound guidance, thus obviating the need for ionizing radiation and iodinated contrast which are potentially deleterious to the patient and operator. The cannulation zone of an avf created with the Ellipsys procedure is typically the upper arm cephalic vein but may be the basilic vein or a brachial vein following transposition to a superficial location [7].

The WavelinQ EndoAVF System incorporates two 4 French catheters. The venous catheter carries a leaf spring Radiofrequency (RF) electrode. The arterial catheter has a ceramic backstop. These two catheters are mated magnetically under fluoroscopic guidance. Once properly mated and aligned, the electrode is energized via a radiofrequency (RF) generator, which is essentially a Bovie electrocautery device set on cutting. This creates a tract fistula as compared to a true tissue weld as is the case of the Ellipsys TRAD device. An arm restraint is utilized to prevent biceps muscle contraction while the electrode is energized. Coil embolization of draining veins is performed at the time of fistula creation. Additional coil embolization and superficialization are performed subsequently as needed.

Clinical Data

Both the Ellipsys and WavelinQ procedures have been evaluated in a modest number of clinical studies. At the time of this writing, results of the Ellipsys procedure have been reported in four clinical studies. Two of these are retrospective studies [8, 9]. Two are prospective studies [6, 10]. The largest and most significant study of the Ellipsys device is the Pivotal trial which will be described in some detail [10].

The Pivotal Trial was a prospective, single-arm study incorporating five sites and enrolling 107 patients. All patients had a proximal radial artery to perforator vein fistula created using the Ellipsys device. The primary endpoints were brachial artery blood flow of greater than or equal to 500 ml/min, a target vein diameter of greater than or equal to 4 mm in greater than 49% of patients, and an absence of complications at 90 days.

Two hundred and sixty-one patients were referred for avf creation. One hundred seventeen (45%) met inclusion criteria. One hundred forty-four patients were excluded from Ellipsys avf creation. Thirteen (5%) were candidates for surgical fistula creation at the wrist. Seventy-three (28%), had unsuitable anatomy. Thus, 72% of referred patients had suitable anatomy for Ellipsys fistula creation.

Ultimately, Ellipsys fistula creation was performed in 102 patients. The target outflow vein was most often the upper arm cephalic vein (74%). The upper arm basilic vein accounted for 24% and the brachial vein 2%.

Maturation and secondary procedures were required in most patients. Anastomotic angioplasty was performed in 72% (77), brachial vein embolization was performed in 32% (34), cubital vein ligation was performed in 31% (33), and surgical transposition was performed in 26% (28).

In terms of results, flow and diameter endpoints were achieved in 86% (92/107). Two-needle dialysis was performed in 88% of patients (71/81) at a mean of 114 ± 66 days.

Functional patencies were 98.4% at 90 days, 98.4% at 180 days, and 92.3% at 1 year.

Early thrombosis (before 30 days) occurred in 12%. This is comparable to the thrombosis rate of 11% that was encountered in the often-cited DAC study, which looked at av. fistula creation in a population of patients treated with clopidogrel [11]. Other complications occurred with the following percentages: late thrombosis in 4%, anastomotic stenosis in 21%, fistula stenosis 16%, steal syndrome 1%. No occurrences of anastomotic pseudoaneurysm were reported.

The authors conclude that Ellipsys is a safe and effective technique for av. fistula creation with results that are comparable to and may be superior to surgical av. fistula creation. In a follow-up study, Beathard et al. reported a 24-month cumulative patency of 92.7% for avf created utilizing the Ellipsys technique [9].

There have been four major clinical studies of the WavelinQ procedure [12–15]. Two of these are retrospective studies [12, 13]. There have been two prospective studies, the NEAT Trial [14] and the EASE Trial [15]. The EASE Trial describes experience with the 4 French WavelinQ system, which is an improved, lower profile version of the device. The original WavelinQ system was 6 French.

The EASE Trial was a prospective single-arm, single-center, multi-operator trial performed in Paraguay. A total of 32 patients were enrolled and had an endo-AVF created using the 4 Fr WavelinQ device. Follow-up was 6 months. Primary endpoints of the study were procedural success, maturation, cannulation success, intervention rate, and patency.

Looking at results, there were no device related events. The anatomy of the endo-AVF created were radial artery to radial vein in 20, and ulnar artery to ulnar vein in the remaining 12. Vessels at the wrist were utilized for the arterial catheter in 72% of cases (23/32), and for the venous catheter in 59% (19/32). The arterial access sites were the radial artery in 59%, brachial artery in 28%, and the ulnar artery in 13%. The venous access site was a distal radial vein in 53%, distal brachial vein in 41%, and distal ulnar vein in 6%.

Technical success was achieved in all study subjects. The adverse event rate was 3% (1/32). This consisted of a venous guidewire vessel perforation which was treated with a stent graft. Primary patency at 6 months was 83%. Cumulative patency at 6 months was 87%. The intervention rate was 0.21 procedures/patient-year.

Physiologic suitability was defined as a fistula with flow greater than 500 ml/min, and a diameter greater than 4 mm. This was achieved in 91% (29/32) by 90 days. Successful 2-needle cannulation was achieved in 78% (21/27) by 90 days. The mean time to cannulation was 43 ± 14 days. Functional cannulation, defined as 2-needle cannulation for 2/3 of sessions/1 month was achieved in 95% (20/21).

The authors conclude that the 4F WavelinQ System is a safe and effective method of endo-AVF creation and that multiple possible access approaches make this a versatile technology.

Important questions remain unanswered by these single-arm studies. These questions include the relative superiority of endo-AVF versus open av. fistula creation and whether there are important differences between the results of the Ellipsys and WavelinQ techniques. To date, there have been no prospective studies to provide a direct comparison of endo-AVF and fistulas created using open surgical techniques. Likewise, there have been no studies that have made a direct comparison of avf created using Ellipsys and WavelinQ. To try and obtain some sense of the relative efficacy of the two endovascular avf techniques, Wee et al. conducted a meta-analysis of the seven major endo-AVF studies [16].

The meta-analysis analyzed the combined results of 300 patients in four WavelinQ and three Ellipsys studies. Technical success was achieved in 97.5%. The 90-day maturation rate was 89.3%. This compares favorably to historical surgical maturation rates of 64–78%. 6-month patency was 91.9% and the 12-month patency was 85.7%.

The complication rate was 5.46%. Unfortunately, secondary interventions were not analyzed due to a lack of data. Only two of the seven studies provided information on secondary interventions. The authors speculate that the secondary intervention rate may be lower than for surgical avf creation. In our experience, secondary interventions are required in the majority of patients receiving an endo-AVF.

Access Planning in the Age of Endo-AVF

Faced with new options for av. access creation, the thoughtful clinician needs to utilize an algorithmic approach that considers the patients' anatomical suitability for both surgical av. fistula creation as well as endo-AVF creation. The decision tree is also influenced by the status of third-party reimbursement, and allowable sites-of-service. Local coverage policies for endo-AVF vary widely by geographic region and carrier.

As of this writing, the New York Medicare-Administrative Contractor (MAC) reimburses for the Ellipsys procedure when performed in a hospital setting or ASC. Ellipsys is not currently a Medicare covered service when performed in the office setting. This is unfortunate, as the procedure can readily be performed in an outpatient setting, which would potentially be of great benefit to the patient and physician in terms of efficiency and convenience. It is also important to note that Medicare excludes the endo-AVF procedures for patients that are candidates for surgical distal forearm fistula creation [17].

The WavelinQ procedure is currently not a Medicare covered service in New York, as it is considered experimental. The LCD states "Coverage of the WavelinQ system must await resolution of ongoing safety issues as well as longer-term data" [17].

There are acceptable minimal anatomic criteria for endo-AVF creation. The proximal radial or proximal ulnar artery should have a diameter of 2 mm and should not have significant calcification. The perforator vein should also have a diameter of at least 2 mm and must be in continuity with the upper arm cephalic, basilic or brachial veins. For the Ellipsys procedure, the perforator vein must be sufficiently non-tortuous that it can be navigated by the straight 21-gauge needle under ultrasound guidance.

Screening for Anatomic Feasibility

In terms of the general applicability of these procedures, it is important to know how often patients present with anatomy suitable for creation of an endo-AVF. In the WavelinQ NEAT Study 75% (132/183) of screened subjects met criteria [14]. In the *Ellipsys* Pivotal trial 72% of subjects achieved "anatomic suitability" [10]. The Ellipsys Post-Market Registry found that 49% (60/123) vein mapped patients were anatomically eligible [7]. In contrast, a much lower incidence of anatomic suitability was reported by Mallios. He found that once patients who could have a radio-cephalic fistula were excluded, 25% of subjects could have an endo-AVF created [8]. This figure is consistent with our anecdotal experience.

Conclusions

The new endo-AVF technologies hold great promise. Potential benefits include minimization of incision and scarring, high patient satisfaction, and increased distal cannulation length. Theorized benefits include a lower risk of aneurysmal degeneration and steal related to lower access pressure and flow consequent to the use of the proximal radial or proximal ulnar artery inflow [18]. There may be a lower intervention rate to achieve maturation, although this has not been definitively demonstrated. Short-term outcomes appear to be comparable to surgical avf, and there may be improved long-term patency. Head-to-head studies are needed to demonstrate the relative merits of the Ellipsys versus WavelinQ procedure, and of fistulas created utilizing the endo-AVF principle versus those created using traditional surgical techniques.

References

1. Brescia MJ, Cimino JE, Appel K, Hurwich BJ. Chronic hemodialysis using venipuncture and a surgically created arteriovenous fistula. N Engl J Med. 1966;275(20):1089–92.
2. Jennings WC, Taubman KE. Alternative autogenous arteriovenous hemodialysis access options. Semin Vasc Surg. 2011;24(2):72–81.
3. Gefen JY, Fox D, Giangola G, Ewing DR, Meisels IS. The transposed forearm loop arteriovenous fistula: a valuable option for primary hemodialysis access in diabetic patients. Ann Vasc Surg. 2002;16(1):89–94.
4. Wasse H, Alvarez AC, Brouwer-Maier D, Hull JE, Balamuthusamy S, Litchfield TF, Cooper RI, Rajan DK, Niyyar VD, Agarwal AK, Abreo K, Lok CE, Jennings WC. Patient selection, education, and cannulation of percutaneous arteriovenous fistulae: an ASDIN white paper. J Vasc Access. 2020;21(6):810–7.
5. Wasse H. Place of percutaneous fistula devices in contemporary management of vascular access. Clin J Am Soc Nephrol. 2019;14(6):938–40.
6. Hull JE, Elizondo-Riojas G, Bishop W, Voneida-Reyna YL. Thermal resistance anastomosis device for the percutaneous creation of arteriovenous fistulae for hemodialysis. J Vasc Interv Radiol. 2017;28(3):380–7.
7. Hull J, Deitrick J, Groome K. Maturation for hemodialysis in the Ellipsys post-market registry. J Vasc Interv Radiol. 2020;31(9):1373–81.
8. Mallios A, Jennings WC, Boura B, Costanzo A, Bourquelot P, Combes M. Early results of percutaneous arteriovenous fistula creation with the Ellipsys vascular access system. J Vasc Surg. 2018;68(4):1150–6.
9. Beathard GA, Litchfield T, Jennings WC. Two-year cumulative patency of endovascular arteriovenous fistula. J Vasc Access. 2020;21(3):350–6.
10. Hull JE, Jennings WC, Cooper RI, Waheed U, Schaefer ME, Narayan R. The pivotal multicenter trial of ultrasound-guided percutaneous arteriovenous fistula creation for hemodialysis access. J Vasc Interv Radiol. 2018;29(2):149–58.
11. Dember LM, Beck GJ, Allon M, Delmez JA, Dixon BS, Greenberg A, Himmelfarb J, Vazquez MA, Gassman JJ, Greene T, Radeva MK, Braden GL, Ikizler TA, Rocco MV, Davidson IJ, Kaufman JS, Meyers CM, Kusek JW, Feldman HI, Dialysis Access Consortium Study Group. Effect of clopidogrel on early failure of arteriovenous fistulas for hemodialysis: a randomized controlled trial. JAMA. 2008;299(18):2164–71.
12. Rajan DK, Ebner A, Desai SB, Rios JM, Cohn WE. Percutaneous creation of an arteriovenous fistula for hemodialysis access. J Vasc Interv Radiol. 2015;26(4):484–90.
13. Radosa CG, Radosa JC, Weiss N, Schmidt C, Werth S, Hofmockel T, Plodeck V, Gatzweiler C, Laniado M, Hoffmann RT. Endovascular creation of an arteriovenous fistula (endoAVF) for hemodialysis access: first results. Cardiovasc Intervent Radiol. 2017;40(10):1545–51.
14. Lok CE, Rajan DK, Clement J, Kiaii M, Sidhu R, Thomson K, Buldo G, Dipchand C, Moist L, Sasal J, NEAT Investigators. Endovascular proximal forearm arteriovenous fistula for hemodi-

alysis access: results of the prospective, multicenter novel endovascular access trial (NEAT). Am J Kidney Dis. 2017;70(4):486–97.
15. Berland TL, Clement J, Griffin J, Westin GG, Ebner A. Endovascular creation of arteriovenous fistulae for hemodialysis access with a 4 Fr device: clinical experience from the EASE study. Ann Vasc Surg. 2019;60:182–92.
16. Yan Wee IJ, Yap HY, Tang TY, Chong TT. A systematic review, meta-analysis, and meta-regression of the efficacy and safety of endovascular arteriovenous fistula creation. J Vasc Surg. 2020;71(1):309–17.
17. Centers for Medicare & Medicaid Services. Local coverage determination (LCD): percutaneous arteriovenous fistula (pAVF) for hemodialysis (L38573). Centers for Medicare & Medicaid Services. 12/03/2020. https://www.cms.gov/medicare-coverage-database/details/lcd-details.aspx?LCDId=38573&ver=8&Cntrctr=341&CntrctrSelected=341*1&name=Noridian+Healthcare+Solutions%2C+LLC+(Noridian+Healthcare+Solutions%2C+LLC+(03301%2C+A+and+B+MAC%2C+J+-+F))&LCntrctr=341*1&DocType=4&bc=AACAAAAAAAAA&.
18. Hebibi H, Achiche J, Franco G, Rottembourg J. Clinical hemodialysis experience with percutaneous arteriovenous fistulas created using the Ellipsys® vascular access system. Hemodial Int. 2019;23(2):167–72.

Chapter 12
Delaying the Onset and Progression of CKD in People with Diabetes: Technology and Effectiveness in Achieving Glucose Control

Alaa Kubbar, Hussam Alkaissi, and Mary Ann Banerji

Introduction

The global prevalence of diabetes is increasing and is a major contributor to the development of kidney disease. In the USA 15% of the adult population has chronic kidney disease; 44% of patients with end-stage kidney disease requiring dialysis were diagnosed with diabetic nephropathy and 25% in European registries of ESRD had diabetes [1, 2]. Among patients with diabetes 37% have chronic kidney disease [3]. Hyperglycemia is the defining abnormality in diabetes and whether established diabetic kidney disease can be completely reversed or only prevented with meticulous treatment of hyperglycemia is still debated. An early proof of concept in type 1 diabetes, showed that pancreas transplantation, providing *prolonged* optimization of blood sugar, may reverse pathological changes of diabetic nephropathy. Structural improvements were not seen at 5 years but only 10 years after pancreas transplantation [4]. The important concept is that improvement in diabetic nephropathy requires a long time and *near normal* glucose control, conditions which have not been matched in 40 years of standard clinical care. Our hope is that the currently evolving technology in insulin sensing and delivery may provide near normal glucose control *early* in the course of diabetes to prevent or slow the progression of kidney and other diabetes complications and possibly improve outcomes in established CKD.

A. Kubbar · H. Alkaissi · M. A. Banerji (✉)
SUNY Downstate Medical Center, Brooklyn, NY, USA
e-mail: Hussam.alkaisi@downstate.edu; MaryAnn.banerji@downstate.edu

S. J. Saggi, M. O. Salifu (eds.), *Technological Advances in Care of Patients with Kidney Diseases*, https://doi.org/10.1007/978-3-031-11942-2_12

CKD in Diabetes and Mortality

In addition to being associated with progressive renal disease, the presence of CKD or ESRD is associated with increased mortality and hospitalizations throughout the spectrum of renal insufficiency [5]. The relationship of complications with glycemic control in ESRD has been controversial because of many confounders including reliability of the hemoglobin A1c a key measure of time integrated glycemic control. Nevertheless, the A1c is the most validated marker of complications. In 23,618 patients on chronic hemodialysis, after adjusting for relevant variables, higher A1c levels (>10%) were associated with increased all-cause and CV mortality [6]. Similarly, a meta-analysis of over 83,000 hemodialysis patients, showed that after adjusting for confounders, a high baseline and mean A1c level (>8.5%) were both significantly associated with increased mortality compared to a lower A1c (6.5–7.4%) [7]. Among participants with high cardiovascular risk, lesser degrees of CKD (stage I–III) are also associated with increased CV risk [8].

The relationship of glucose to diabetes complications in ESRD is poorly understood because most glucose lowering trials excluded patients with advanced and end-stage renal disease (ESRD) as achieving stable glucose control is frequently challenging. The management of diabetes in CKD is complicated by many metabolic changes including increased insulin resistance, impaired glucose metabolism, increased hepatic gluconeogenesis, failure of renal gluconeogenesis, decreased insulin clearance, and increased red blood cell glucose uptake during hemodialysis and impaired counter-regulatory hormones including growth hormone and cortisol. These changes amplify any tendencies to glycemic dysregulation, and both hypoglycemia and hyperglycemia are common. Ultimately, decreased insulin clearance and renal gluconeogenesis conspire to increase hypoglycemia.

Role of Glycemic Control in Preventing the Progression of CKD

Although most clinical trials of glucose lowering treatments on decreasing complications excluded patients with significant CKD, major randomized trials, described below have addressed the primary and secondary prevention of *early* CKD and inform our approaches to slowing its development.

One of the major randomized control trials, the Diabetes Control and Complications Trial (DCCT) in early Type 1 diabetes demonstrated a clear decrease in the progression of microvascular disease including nephropathy and retinopathy [9]. In type 2 diabetes, the outcomes are less clear, possibly as the numbers of events are low and the duration of follow-up is not long enough. A patient level meta-analysis showed that more intensive glucose control compared to less, led to significant 20% risk reductions in composite ESRD, renal death and development of an estimated GFR (eGFR) < 30 ml/min and development of macroalbuminuria

[10–14]. The median follow-up of these studies were 5 years and included the UK Prospective Diabetes Study (UKPDS), Action to Control Cardiovascular Risk in Diabetes (ACCORD), Action in Diabetes and Vascular Disease (ADVANCE) trial, and Veterans Affairs Diabetes Trial (VADT) [10–14]. In terms of mortality, the results were conflicting. DCCT and UKPDS trials showed no effect on mortality at the end of the trials but long-term data at follow-up showed significant reduction in participants who had been in the intensive glycemic control group despite similar glycemic control during the follow-up period. There was no difference in mortality in the ADVANCE and VADT trials, though the ACCORD trial showed higher mortality with intensive glucose control. Patient level meta-analysis of the four major trials of type 2 diabetes with a mean treatment duration of 4.4 years, showed a modest (HR 0.91), but significant reduction in cardiovascular mortality with a significant 15% reduction in myocardial infarction, no reduction in all-cause mortality and a significant increase in hypoglycemia (HR 2.48) [6]. Post-hoc analyses showed that in the ACCORD study of patients with high CV risk who had mild CKD (I–III), intensive glycemic treatment led to an increase all-cause and CV mortality (HR 1.31 and 1.41, respectively) [8], suggesting that intensive glycemic control in CKD may require less intense glycemic targets and improved monitoring of blood sugars. A key concept is that while there are glycemic benefits with short-term intensive glucose control, longer studies of sustained glycemic control without hypoglycemia will be required to demonstrate this benefit.

It is clear that the complications and mortality of diabetes are not solely mitigated by glucose control. This was demonstrated in the STENO 2 trial which provided intensive multifactorial treatment including glucose and lipid lowering, renin-angiotensin blockers, and aspirin [15]. This study was relatively small but of a longer duration in type 2 diabetes who had persistent microalbuminuria (a risk factor for both kidney and vascular complications). Patients were studied for mean of 7.8 years, then observed for a mean of 5.5 years. At 4 and 8 years of treatment, nephropathy and retinopathy decreased by ~40% in the intensive group but a 50% decrease in mortality did not occur until 10 years of multifactorial intensive treatment. At the end of the 13 years, the STENO 2 trial results demonstrated decreased mortality, nephropathy, retinopathy, peripheral neuropathy, and autonomic neuropathy. The difference in glucose lowering of an A1c of 0.5% was modest at best but the long duration combined with a multifactorial approach form the basis of our current practice for preventing complications. This highlights the duration of improved plasma glucose required for structural changes to become manifest.

Thus, early interventions in optimizing glucose control are essential to both prevent diabetic nephropathy and reverse the *early changes* of diabetic nephropathy. The technologies described below are likely to play an important role in achieving this. Other targets for intervention, especially when chronic kidney disease is established, include lipid, blood pressure, renin-angiotensin system, and inflammation. Because ESRD is not common and takes a long time to develop, long-term studies are needed. Precision medicine may identify individuals who are particularly responsive glucose lowering while others may require a different focus, including the use SGLT2-inhibitors and as yet undiscovered approaches.

Technology in the Prevention of Diabetic Kidney Disease

As mentioned earlier, intensive glucose-lowering therapy has been associated with lower microvascular complications, including diabetic nephropathy, yet some significant trials showed conflicting data on mortality. Intensive glucose-lowering therapy aims for lower HbA1c goals and is invariably associated with hypoglycemia, an archenemy of the diabetologist and the rate limiting step for optimizing glucose control.

The hemoglobin A1c is the gold standard surrogate marker of glycemic control and predicts microvascular outcomes. Yet, it is a single average of glucose fluctuations over approximately 3 months, making it difficult to use as a decision tool for day-to-day treatment. People with diabetes experience fluctuation in glucose levels during the day, referred to as "glucose excursion." The HbA1c does not reflect these fluctuations; two patients may have the same HbA1c value, one with stable glucose levels around the mean and one with large troughs and valleys around the mean.

One way to address this discrepancy is by examining "time in range." Time in range has been defined as the percentage time of the day when glucose levels are within set limits of 70–180 mg/dl (7.8–10 mmol/l) and is increasingly being accepted as a useful and validated management tool by both physicians and patients.

With the standard measurement of 1–4 daily blood glucose levels using the capillary blood sample, the small number of data points are generated make it challenging to maintain a good time in range or TIR. However, with advances such as continuous glucose monitoring (CGM) data points can be obtained virtually every 5 min up to 288 times/day. The CGM has a catheter inserted into the subcutaneous tissue through which glucose is measured continuously and transmitted locally to a sensor for a real-time read-out and a timely response by the patient. When the CGM is connected to a closed-loop insulin pump, with decisions can be made in real-time to alter insulin delivery based on glucose levels. This permits optimizing the time in range and the maintenance of a lower HbA1c with a lower risk of hypoglycemia, with lesser glycemic excursions (or variations around mean of glucose levels). Consensus conferences of national and international societies have supported the early use of this technology [16].

The time in range measure derived from the CGM was recently validated as associated with 8-year progression of microvascular outcomes including retinopathy and nephropathy (microalbuminuria). Using seven point capillary blood glucose testing results, a time in range profile was created from the Diabetes Control and Complications Trial (DCCT) in Type 1 diabetes which was originally published in 1993. Beck et al. found that for each 10% drop in "time in range," there was an increased hazard rate for developing microalbuminuria (moderately increased albuminuria) of 40% and a 64% increased risk of retinopathy [17]. The DCCT was the pivotal study to validate the HbA1c as a target for treatment and now has validated the time in range or TIR. This metric is being increasingly accepted as being useful for guiding therapy for patients interested in proactively decreasing complications.

CGM can be paired with either an insulin pump or self-injected for insulin delivery. With either insulin delivery approach, the patient decides on the number of units or dose of insulin required, either with meals or as correction; this had been referred to as *sensor-augmented pump*. Newer pumps are supplemented with algorithm that can alter insulin delivery based on glucose levels in real time, without the need of human intervention, and this had been referred to as a *closed-loop system*, aka the artificial pancreas.

In the iDCL trial, Breton et al. used a closed-loop insulin pump compared to a sensor-augmented pump in the control group to examine time in range in children with T1DM [18]. A closed-loop system connected to CGM was associated with a "time in range" of 11% higher time points than the control group. Inspection showed the highest time in range was achieved at early hours of the day, during sleeping. During sleep, we lose conscious control and decision making to correct glucose levels and glucose levels drift to either direction, namely, hypo or hyperglycemia. Interestingly, HbA1c did not differ significantly between the groups, with HbA1c of 7.6% in the closed-loop system and 7.9% in the sensor-adjusted system. Thus, this trial shows the importance of the CGM closed loop in maintaining time in range and shows that two patients with similar HbA1c can have different times in range. We know from Fioretto et al. [4] that to reverse diabetes glomerulopathy, one may need at least 5 and up to 10 years of normoglycemia, and one way to approach this is by increasing time in range using CGM as shown by iDCL trial.

Technology in Established ESRD and Diabetes

To date, CGM has not yet been approved by the FDA for use in ESRD patients treated with hemodialysis. Optimal glycemic control may reduce morbidity and mortality in these patients, but it is difficult to achieve because of the alternation between dialysis and non-dialysis periods. Kepenekian et al. conducted a prospective multicenter study analyzing 28 hemodialyzed patients with type 2 diabetes treated by a basal-bolus insulin regimen responsive to CGM glucose values over 3 months. Results demonstrated that HbA1c significantly decreased from 8.4 ± 1.0% to 7.6 ± 1.0% ($p < 0.01$). Similarly, mean CGM glucose values significantly decreased from 9.9 ± 1.9 to 8.9 ± 2.1 mmol/L ($p = 0.05$). The frequency of hyperglycemia significantly decreased from 41.3 ± 21.9% to 30.1 ± 22.4% ($p < 0.05$), without a significant increase in hypoglycemia. They concluded that CGM improves glycemic control without increasing hypoglycemic events or weight gain in hemodialyzed diabetic patients [19].

The DIALYDIAB trial reported on the effectiveness of CGM in hemodialysis patients with diabetes on decreasing HbA1c [20]. A total of 15 dialysis patients were studied over 12 weeks and assessed by self-monitoring blood glucose three times per day during 6 weeks, followed by a 5-day CGM recording at a 2-week interval for another 6 weeks. Glucose values were sent to a diabetes expert who proposed changes in the anti-diabetes drugs. This pilot study found that the mean

CGM glucose at baseline was 8.3 ± 2.5 mmol/l, and unchanged at 8.2 ± 1.6 mmol/l after SBGM but significantly lower at 7.7 ± 1.6 mmol/l compared to baseline. The A1c decreased significantly from 6.85 to 6.46 while using CGM. Treatment regimens were more frequently changed during CGM use and glycemic levels were lower on dialysis days. Like Kepenekian [19], in hemodialysis patients, CGM monitoring was associated with better glucose control without increased risk of hypoglycemia.

More recently, in 2018, Yeoh et al. compared the efficacy of self-monitoring of blood glucose (SMBG) versus *retrospective CGM* in improving glycemic control in DKD stage 3. They randomized 30 patients with DKD on anti-diabetic agents and compared their HbA1c and hypoglycemia incidence. Results showed that HbA1c improved significantly from baseline 9.9 ± 1.2 to 9.0 ± 1.5% ($p < 0.001$) at 3 months, within each group with no difference between CGM or SMBG groups. However, in the CGM group, the percentage duration in hyperglycemia reduced from baseline 65.4 ± 22.4% to 54.6 ± 23.6% ($p = 0.033$) at 6 weeks, with a non-significant rise in percentage duration in hypoglycemia from 1.2 ± 2.2% to 4.0 ± 7.0% ($p = 0.176$). There was no difference in self-reported and documented hypoglycemia events. Short-term episodic use of CGM reduced time spent in the hyperglycemia range without significantly increasing hypoglycemia [20, 21].

These studies are small and will require confirmation in larger studies and links with improved outcomes.

In summary, intensive glucose-lowering therapy in people with diabetes decreases microvascular complications, including nephropathy. Therefore, prevention of CKD development and progression should begin with adequate glucose management and maintained for long durations. Although the optimal approach to glycemic control in patients with type 2 diabetes and advanced CKD remains unclear, evidence supports individualization of treatment. CGM use has the advantage of providing a better assessment of glycemic patterns and insulin needs among diabetic patients with advanced CKD. Pilot studies have shown that CGM use in patients with CKD and ESRD on hemodialysis improves glycemic control and reduces time spent in the hyperglycemia range without significantly increasing exposure to hypoglycemia. Moreover, CGM can recognize declining glucose levels before the occurrence of hypoglycemia, which could be life-saving for these patients. Thus, CGM has the potential to become a new gold standard for the assessment of glycemic control in diabetic patients treated by hemodialysis, especially given the known limitations of HbA1c and other glycemic biomarkers and their propensity for hypoglycemia.

References

1. https://www.usrds.org/2019/view/USRDS_2019_ES_final.pdf. Accessed 20 Nov 2021.
2. https://www.era-edta-reg.org/files/annualreports/pdf/AnnRep2016.pdf. Accessed 20 Nov 2021.
3. Weir MR. Chronic kidney disease and type 2 diabetes. An American Diabetes Association monograph. 2021. https://professional.diabetes.org.

4. Fioretto P, Steffes MW, Sutherland DE, Goetz FC, Mauer M. Reversal of lesions of diabetic nephropathy after pancreas transplantation. N Engl J Med. 1998;339:69–75.
5. Go AS, Chertow GM, Fan D, McCulloch CE, Hsu C. Chronic kidney disease and the risks of death, cardiovascular events, and hospitalization. N Engl J Med. 2004;351:1296–305.
6. Kalanter-Zadeh K, Aronowitz J, Kopple JD, et al. A1C and survival in maintenance hemodialysis patients. Diab Care. 2007;30:1049–55.
7. Hill CJ, Maxwell AP, Cardwell CR, et al. Glycated hemoglobin and risk of death in diabetic patients treated with hemodialysis: a meta-analysis. Am J Kidney Dis. 2014;63:84–94.
8. Papademetriou V, Loveto L, Doumas M, Nylen E, Mottl A, Cohen R, et al. Chronic kidney disease and intensive glycemic control increase CV risk in patient with type 2 diabetes. Kidney Int. 2015;87:649–59.
9. Ohkubo Y, Kishikawa H, Araki E, Miyata T, Isami S, Motoyoshi S, Kojima Y, Furuyoshi N, Shichiri M. Intensive insulin therapy prevents the progression of diabetic microvascular complications in Japanese patients with non-insulin-dependent diabetes mellitus: a randomized prospective 6-year study. Diabetes Res Clin Pract. 1995;28:103–17. https://doi.org/10.1016/0168-8227(95)01064-k.
10. Nathan D, Genuth S, Lachin J, et al. Diabetes control and complications trial research group: the effect of intensive treatment of diabetes on the development and progression of long-term complications in insulin-dependent diabetes mellitus. N Engl J Med. 1993;329:977–86.
11. Patel A, MacMahon S, Chalmers J, et al. Intensive glucose control and vascular outcomes in patients with type 2 diabetes. N Engl J Med. 2008;358:2560–72.
12. Ismail-Beigi F, Craven T, Banerji MA, et al. Effect of intensive treatment of hyperglycemia on microvascular outcomes in type 2 diabetes: an analysis of the ACCORD randomized trial. Lancet. 2010;376:419–30.
13. Duckworth W, Abraira C, Moritz T, et al. Glucose control and vascular complications in veterans with type 2 diabetes. N Engl J Med. 2009;360:129–39.
14. Zoungas S, Arima H, Gerstein HC, et al., The Collaborators on Trials of Lowering Glucose (CONTROL) group. Effects of intensive glucose control on microvascular outcomes in patients with type 2 diabetes: a meta-analysis of individual participant data from randomized controlled trials. Lancet Diabetes Endocrinol. 2017; 5(6):431–37. https://doi.org/10.1016/S2213-8587(17)30104-3.
15. Gaede P, Lund-Andersen H, Parving H-H, Pedersen O. Effect of a multifactorial intervention on mortality in type 2 diabetes. N Engl J Med. 2008;358:580–91.
16. Danne T, Nimri R, Battelino T, et al. International consensus on use of continuous glucose monitoring. Diabetes Care. 2017;40:1631–40.
17. Beck RW, Bergenstal RM, Riddlesworth TD, Kollman C, Li Z, Brown AS, Close KL. Validation of time in range as an outcome measure for diabetes clinical trials. Diabetes Care. 2019;42:400–5. https://doi.org/10.2337/dc18-1444.
18. Breton MD, Kanapka LG, Beck RW, Ekhlaspour L, Forlenza GP, Cengiz E, Schoelwer M, Ruedy KJ, Jost E, Carria L, et al. A randomized trial of closed-loop control in children with type 1 diabetes. N Engl J Med. 2020;383:836–45.
19. Kepenekian L, Smagala A, Meyer L, et al. Continuous glucose monitoring in hemodialyzed patients with type 2 diabetes: a multicenter pilot study. Clin Nephrol. 2014;82:240–6.
20. Joubert M, Fourmy C, Henri P, Ficheux M, Lobbedez T, Reznik Y. Effectiveness of continuous glucose monitoring in dialysis patients with diabetes: the DIALYDIAB pilot study. Diabetes Res Clin Pract. 2015;107:348–54. https://doi.org/10.1016/j.diabres.2015.01.026.
21. Yeoh E, Lim BK, Fun S, Tong J, Yeoh LY, Sum CF, Subramaniam T, Lim SC. Efficacy of self-monitoring of blood glucose versus retrospective continuous glucose monitoring in improving glycaemic control in diabetic kidney disease patients. Nephrology (Carlton). 2018;23:264–8. https://doi.org/10.1111/nep.12978.

Chapter 13
Strategies and Technologies to Advance Kidney Health from Kidney Health Initiative

Errol Carter, Subodh J. Saggi, and Moro O. Salifu

Strategies and Technologies to Advance Kidney Health from Kidney Health Initiative

Over the years, we have seen advancements in kidney care but the recent executive order for "Advancing American Kidney Health" [1] has supercharged the effort. With strategies designed to

- Prevent kidney failure whenever possible through better diagnosis, treatment, and incentives for preventive care.
- Increase patient choice through affordable alternative treatments for ESRD by encouraging higher value care, educating patients on treatment alternatives, and development of artificial kidneys.
- "Increase access to kidney transplants by modernizing the organ recovery and transplantation systems and updating regulations" [2].

The order has inspired a level of technological innovation in the industry. "In 2012, the American Society of Nephrology and the US Food and Drug Administration (FDA) established a public-private partnership (with the intension of infusing innovation and development of effective new therapies for people with kidney disease. Industry partners such as dialysis providers, pharmaceutical companies, research institutions, patient organizations, device manufacturers, foundations, health

E. Carter (✉)
Medicine, SUNY Downstate Health Sciences University, Brooklyn, NY, USA

Adjunct Faculty-CUNY Queensborough Community College, Bayside, NY, USA
e-mail: Errol.Carter@downstate.edu

S. J. Saggi · M. O. Salifu
Medicine, SUNY Downstate Health Sciences University, Brooklyn, NY, USA
e-mail: subodh.saggi@downstate.edu; moro.salifu@downstate.edu

S. J. Saggi, M. O. Salifu (eds.), *Technological Advances in Care of Patients with Kidney Diseases*, https://doi.org/10.1007/978-3-031-11942-2_13

professional organizations and government agencies, came together to form the Kidney Health Initiative" [3, 4]. This led to the creation of the Kidney Innovation Accelerator (Kidney X), the organization leading the drive behind new technologies and therapeutics.

To inspire innovation, Kidney X instituted a Redesign Dialysis competition. The ideas and solutions generated by this competition are numerous, varied and broken out in two categories. "The first category looked at solutions that are already tried or put into practice. Category two where we've seen some ground-breaking ideas, look at ideas for solutions not yet created" [5]. A variety are listed on the Kidney X website. A small sample is listed here.

Patient Innovator Challenge Winners

- *Category 1.*
  - App to monitor blood test results.
  - A way to extend the life of a kidney removed for transplantation to give surgeons more time to access the organ.
  - Creating kidney patient diet booklets geared toward patient cultural cuisine.
  - Creating a device to monitor fluid levels in dialysis patients.
  - A device that disinfects tubing for peritoneal dialysis.
  - A device to help a one-handed veteran administer home dialysis.
  - A 3D-printable wrist cuff to secure needles used in home dialysis.
  - Using a state-funded home aide program to hire someone to help with home dialysis.
  - Creating clothing suited for dialysis patients.
  - A video cooking series for end-stage kidney failure patients.
- *Category 2*
  - A Bioresorbable Shape Memory Polymer Wrap to Improve Maturation and Patency of Dialysis Access Sites.
  - A Novel Device to Prevent Infection Due to Touch Contamination in Peritoneal Dialysis.
  - A Pro-Regenerative Vascular Access Graft.
  - Intracorporeal Hemodialysis System (iHemo).
  - Developing Self-Renewable "Living" Endothelium Vascular Grafts for Hemodialysis.
  - Nitric Oxide-Eluting, Disposable Hemodialysis Catheter Cap to Prevent Infection and Thrombosis" [5–7].

This government led effort has sparked movement in the industry and is producing innovations that can change how kidney failure is combatted in the future. "In the past, manufacturers and providers have implemented changes that have improved patients lives, however, these improvements were geared towards the current kidney replacement therapies that have seen little change over decades. There is a reluctance to invest in innovative products as long as companies can profit from current technologies while growth in the market is still promising and research and development comes at a high cost" [8]. Although this is the tendency, these companies and providers still offer technologies that improve the quality of care for their patients. They have embraced President Donald Trump's executive order. There are various new devices and technologies developed and in development. For example, we see some for vascular access, some devices focused on infection control, and others targeting fluid control. One device that we have been using at SUNY Parkside Dialysis, the CLiC™ device that is used with the 2008T machine to noninvasively measure hematocrit, percent change in blood volume and oxygen saturation in real time, is an example of the technology enhancing today's therapeutic methods. Companies are improving on and using new tools for monitoring treatments both in-center and remotely. At SUNY, we have partnered with a company that remotely monitors patients' treatments and provide us with early warnings of pending vascular access problems. Tele-health has become mainstream since the COVID-19 pandemic. Methods designed to increase kidney transplants and increase the number of patients choosing a home modality have also increased. Despite the benefits of these new technologies, methods, and processes, the provision of kidney care remains fundamentally the same.

The exciting new innovations on the horizon will disrupt today's dialysis markets and force changes in how care is administered to patients with kidney failure. Many new technologies being developed would greatly improve the quality of life for patients with kidney disease. There is work being done on wearable, portable, and implantable devices in numerous countries. One such wearable device under development, "a toxin-removal technology named Photo-Oxidation Urea Removal (POUR)" [9], shows great potential. This device would enable dialysis using only a liter of dialysate. "A portable blood-purification device called QIDNI/D" [10] is hoping to start human trials in 2022. These devices all aim to give patients more freedom and flexibility in their daily lives. The success of these devices would mean that patients are no longer destined to spend countless hours treating in-center or stuck at home connected to bulky machines. The "implantable bioartificial kidney" [11] currently in preclinical development is the device that could ultimately relieve patients from having to rely on dialysis. With the aid of these devices, patients will be able to move about for work and leisure while getting treated. In some cases, treatment would be continuous. It is no wonder that "specialists believe such technology is the promise for the future" [12].

While we await the advent of such new technology, it is good to know that there is continuous improvement on how patients are cared for today. More importantly though, with the anticipated growth in the number of patients who will require dialysis, developing technologies that will bring care to those who were once unable to access care are also progressing. These technologies include enabling "water purification at the point of care" [13] and a "blood-less system that uses a cup of water" [14]. In addition to bringing dialysis to the masses, these technologies will drastically reduce the cost of treatment.

Undoubtedly, the Kidney Health Initiative is driving the industry in the right direction. The ideas, solutions, and developing technologies conceived go from the very simple to the very complex. Optimistically, each has the potential to improve patient care, help to reduce the cost of care, and enhance the quality of life of the kidney disease patient. These patients can look forward to a future where they are no longer saddled to a time exhausting schedule hooked up to dialysis machines and hoping for a transplant. They will be able to go about their lives while focusing on their health care needs.

References

1. HHS launches President Trump's 'Advancing American Kidney Health' initiative. HHS.Gov; 2019. https://www.hhs.gov/about/news/2019/07/10/hhs-launches-president-trump-advancing-american-kidney-health-initiative.html.
2. The White House. Executive order on advancing American Kidney Health [Press release]; 2019, July 10. https://www.whitehouse.gov/presidential-actions/executive-order-advancing-american-kidney-health/.
3. Harris RC, Cahill Z. How the kidney health initiative catalyzes innovation in a dynamic environment. Clin J Am Soc Nephrol. 2019;15(3):421–2. https://doi.org/10.2215/cjn.11060919.
4. U.S. Department of Health and Human Services, Azar II AM. Advancing American Kidney Health; 2019, July. U.S. Department of Health and Human Services. https://aspe.hhs.gov/sites/default/files/migrated_legacy_files//189996/AdvancingAmericanKidneyHealth.pdf.
5. Nesbitt H. KidneyX | Innovation Accelerator. American Society of Nephrology; 2019. https://www.kidneyx.org/.
6. Nesbitt H. Prize winners. American Society of Nephrology; 2019. http://www.kidneyx.org/PrizeCompetitions/PrizeWinners.
7. Nesbitt H. KidneyX | In The News. American Society of Nephrology; 2019. https://www.kidneyx.org/pages/news.aspx.
8. Norton JM, Moxey-Mims MM, Eggers PW, Narva AS, Star RA, Kimmel PL, Rodgers GP. Social determinants of racial disparities in CKD. J Am Soc Nephrol. 2016;27(9):2576–95. https://doi.org/10.1681/asn.2016010027.
9. Antia M. Washington Research Foundation awards $230,052 to Center for Dialysis Innovation researchers to improve in-home dialysis. EIN News; 2021, August 20. https://www.einnews.com/pr_news/549347927/washington-research-foundation-awards-230-052-to-center-for-dialysis-innovation-researchers-to-improve-in-home-dialysis
10. Beutuel E. Mobile dialysis startup eyes human trials in 2022 following encouraging animal study. https://Techcrunch.Com/; 2021, June 17. https://techcrunch.com/2021/06/17/mobile-dialysis-startup-eyes-human-trials-in-2022-following-encouraging-animal-study/?guccounter=1&guce_referrer=aHR0cHM6Ly93d3cuZ29vZ2xlLmNvbS8&guce_referrer_sig=AQAAANjPq_5o_Cpfth3kf8EiMGjitIm1QrcYVzq0Vs7TA-zK3mMskHVgvC7YU2ivuVV0Xh5UY_owmJL6rDL3OLCXosbSMnK_SbS4eueFl4I8Cc_-vNarapjW2VoiEbKkPtspOg1Na7K0PwMFc69v3vC2iL34ZaJr7t6StrxtGSMZZKwf
11. Charnow JA. Progress on an implantable bioartificial kidney. Home » news » nephrology » end-stage renal disease; 2022, April 1. https://www.renalandurologynews.com/home/news/nephrology/end-stage-renal-disease/investigator-provides-update-on-development-of-an-implantable-bioartificial-kidney/. Accessed 15 May 2022.
12. Fortuna G. Promising portable kidney faces innovation, portability bottlenecks. www.Euractiv.Com; 2021, July 14. https://www.euractiv.com/section/health-consumers/news/promising-portable-kidney-faces-innovation-portability-bottlenecks/.

13. Henderson EB. New dialysis system shows ability to make sterile, medical grade water at the point-of-care. News-Medical.Net; 2022, February 28. https://www.news-medical.net/news/20220227/New-dialysis-system-shows-ability-to-make-sterile-medical-grade-water-at-the-point-of-care.aspx#:%7E:text=by%202%20people-,New%20dialysis%20system%20shows%20ability%20to%20make%20sterile%2C%20medical%20grade,at%20the%20point%2Dof%2Dcare&text=Findings%20from%20preliminary%20tests%20of,for%20patients%20with%20kidney%20failure.
14. Tribune. Pakistan develops first bloodless kidney dialysis machine. The Express Tribune; 2021, December 24. https://tribune.com.pk/story/2262202/pakistan-develops-first-bloodless-kidney-dialysis-machine.

Chapter 14
Current Noninvasive Technologies in Interventions to Control Hyperparathyroid Bone Diseases of CKD and ESRD

Satoshi Funakoshi

Introduction

Secondary hyperparathyroidism (SHPT) is a crucial issue among patients on dialysis therapy, as it has a negative impact on the cardiovascular system, chronic kidney disease-mineral, and bone disorders and patient prognosis [1]. To treat this disorder, active vitamin D compounds, alfa-calcidol, paricalcitol or 22-oxacalcitol have been administered to patients on hemodialysis (HD). Moreover, calcimimetics such as cinacalcet attenuate SHPT effectively by allosterically modulating the calcium-sensing receptor on parathyroid glands and augmenting extracellular calcium sensitivity [2].

Parathyroidectomy with auto-transplantation and percutaneous ethanol injection (PEIT) has played an important role in controlling SHPT. Nonetheless, various surgical interventions have significantly decreased after the emerge of calcimimetics [3]. Although the efficacy of calcimimetics has been well recognized, these products could evoke gastrointestinal adverse effects, such as nausea and vomiting, and the cost burden of calcimimetics has become serious in long-term HD [4].

In the past, percutaneous interventions for SHPT are implemented by using ethanol to degenerate parathyroids, but ethanol causes serious necrosis when it leaks outside of parathyroid glands, the application of PEIT became limited use. Subsequently, local injection of active vitamin D was attempted to safely augment the effect of the drugs [5]. Instead of ethanol and active vitamin D, we performed a local injection of etelcalcetide, a new calcimimetics for the treatment of SHPT. Etelcalcetide is composed of seven D-body amino acids (molecular weight 1048 Da) and is not expected to be metabolized by enzymes in the human body. The clearance of etelcalcetide mainly depends on renal excretion. Due to the properties

S. Funakoshi (✉)
Nagasaki Kidney Center, Nagasaki, Japan

S. J. Saggi, M. O. Salifu (eds.), *Technological Advances in Care of Patients with Kidney Diseases*, https://doi.org/10.1007/978-3-031-11942-2_14

of this compound, it is mainly eliminated from dialysis among patients on HD despite reversible disulfide exchange with albumin [6]. Consequently, the direct injection of etelcalcetide in parathyroids could be an activator of the calcium sensing receptor for a certain amount of time, and it is expected to be much safer than ethanol. In this chapter percutaneous injection methods are reviewed, showing the results of our pilot study of local etelcalcetide injection in the parathyroid glands.

Patients and Methods

Ten HD patients with SHPT) who experienced nausea while on cinacalcet or etelcalcetide were enrolled in this study after obtaining their written informed consent. Cinacalcet or etelcalcetide was withdrawn from all patients for >2 weeks before the local injection. Following the Japanese Society for Parathyroid Intervention Guidelines for PEIT [7], etelcalcetide was injected locally under direct real-time ultrasonographic guidance until it permeated through 80% of the estimated parathyroid gland volume. After attaching a bracket to the probe, needle was advance visually using real-time ultrasonographic guidance to determine the location of the tip. After confirming the jet echo within the gland, 1 mL (2.5 mg) of etelcalcetide is injected directly into the parathyroid glands per 1.25 mL of gland volume (Fig. 14.1).

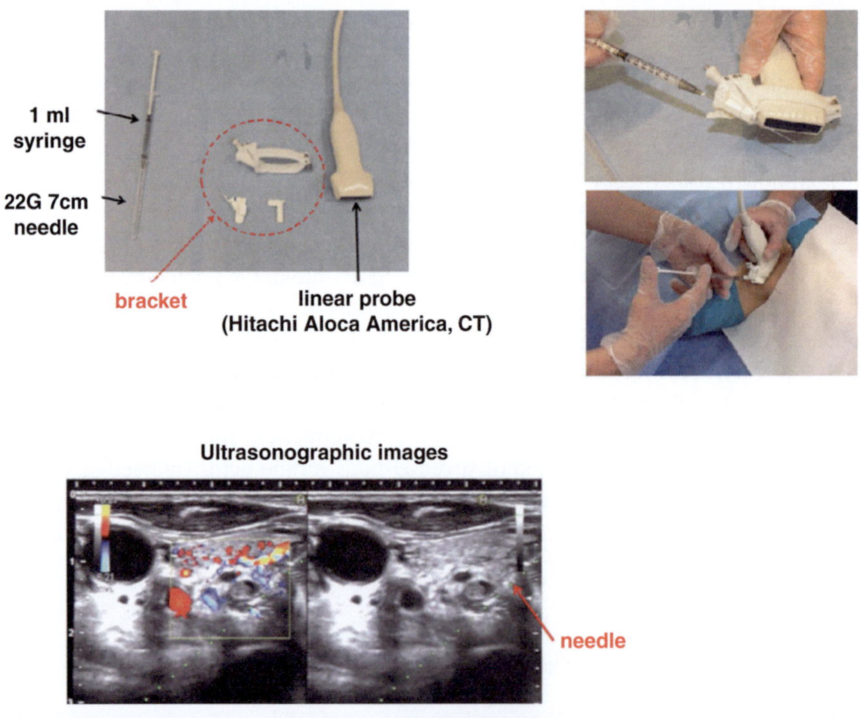

Fig. 14.1 Devices and procedures

To ensure that there were no adverse events, investigators paid careful attention to patients during the local injection.

Serum intact serum parathyroid hormone (iPTH) levels were measured at −4, 0, 1, 2, 4, 6, and 8 weeks. Patients were defined as responders when they achieved a > 50% reduction in iPTH levels. If iPTH increased excessively during this period, systemic administration of etelcalcetide at) 5 mg × 3 per week was initiated as a rescue therapy.

Results

All ten patients (mean age, 67.8 years; median HD duration, 11.8 years) were treated with cinacalcet orally or etelcalcetide intravenously before the local injection of etelcalcetide (Table 14.1).

Five patients achieved a > 50% reduction in serum iPTH level and were defined as responders. Serum iPTH levels remained within 300 pg/mL throughout the study period. In contrast, the remaining five patients did not respond to this therapy ("non-responders") (Fig. 14.2) [8]. Two non-responders were administered an intravenous injection of etelcalcetide 2 weeks after the local injection, and the other three non-responders received an intravenous injection of etelcalcetide 4 weeks after the injection. Serum iPTH levels promptly decreased with the rescue of systemic etelcalcetide administration (Table 14.1).

Although there was no significant difference in the number of enlarged parathyroid glands, the responders had significantly shorter HD vintage, shorter durations of prior cinacalcet treatment, and less accumulated amount of cinacalcet (Table 14.1).

Apart from patient D at 2 weeks and patient J at 2 weeks, there was no significant decline in serum calcium level. The former was 8.4 mg/dL, and the latter was 8.3 mg/dL, respectively. Furthermore, hypocalcemia-related symptoms, such as muscle clamping and paresthesia, were not induced, and hypophosphatemia (−3.5 mg/dL) was not observed during this period. No serious injection-related complications, such as hematoma or laryngeal nerve paresis, were observed.

Table 14.1 The backgrounds of patients who received local injection of etelcalcetide and the transition of iPTH level during the period

	Age	Sex	HD vintage (years)	No. of grands	Cinacalcet treatment (months)	Accumulated amount of cinacalcet (g)	Pre-treatment cinacalcet (mg)	iPTH −4 weeks (pg/mL)	iPTH 0 weeks (pg/mL)	iPTH 1 weeks (pg/mL)	iPTH 2 weeks (pg/mL)	iPTH 4 weeks (pg/mL)	iPTH 6 weeks (pg/mL)	iPTH 8 weeks (pg/mL)
Mean	63.2		8	2.2	30.6	29.0	40	249	267.6	151.6	102.8	115.6	144.8	177.4
A	66	M	12	3	8	6	25	360	359	180	124	57	70	126
B	59	F	7	2	7	14	50	357	346	154	121	141	207	286
C	59	F	7	2	7	14	50	284	323	201	146	196	204	193
D	57	M	9	2	99	60	50	165	218	172	101	153	166	193
E	75	F	5	2	32	50.9	25	79	92	51	22	31	77	89
Mean	72.4		15.6	2	67	76.4	40	197.6	435.2	434.2	407.8			
F	67	M	5	1	45	33.8	25	274	289	373	301	397[a]	244[a]	151[a]
G	77	M	19	2	110	174	50	62	151	168	171	272	260[a]	122[a]
H	73	M	27	2	83	62.3	25	262	256	290	305	199[a]	193[a]	189[a]
I	76	M	16	2	47	74.3	75	221	501	514	543	809	563[a]	282[a]
J	69	M	11	3	50	37.5	25	169	979	826	719	238[a]	236[a]	219[a]

HD hemodialysis, *iPTH* intact para thyroid hormone
[a] Systemic etelcalcetide injection (5 mg × 3 per week)

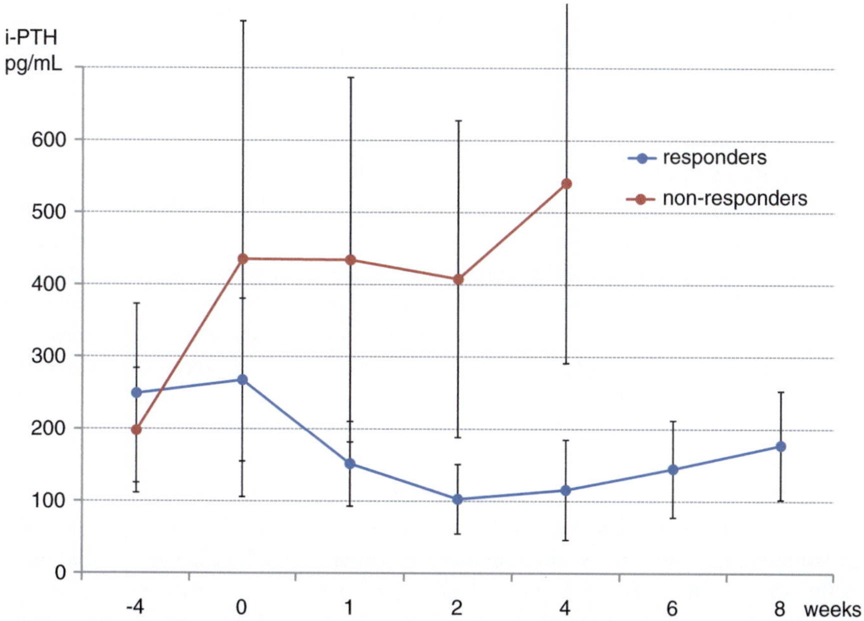

Fig. 14.2 The effects of the direct injection of etelcalcetide in parathyroid grands

Discussion

We carried out a pilot study of local etelcalcetide injection directly into the parathyroid glands in ten patients with secondary hyperparathyroidism who did not tolerate the adverse effects caused by the systemic administration of cinacalcet or etelcalcetide. The procedure of local injection directly into the parathyroid glands requires a high-resolution ultrasound machine, special devices, and skills but costs approximately $10 in one treatment including the etelcalcetide fee. Although there were no complications in this study, only half of the patients achieved successful control of SHPT. The responders tended to have shorter HD vintages, shorter durations, and lower accumulating doses of cinacalcet. The reasons for the difference in response to etelcalcetide injection to the glands remains unclear. Cinacalcet has been reported to reduce parathyroid gland volume [8], but there were no significant differences in the number and size of glands between responders and non-responders in this preliminary trial. We speculate that factors such as changes in the receptor profile to calcimimetics may have been altered after long-term administration of cinacalcet. The administration of cinacalcet could affect calcium-sensing receptor expression [9] and may cause morphological changes in the parathyroid glands, and a qualitative change can occur in the parathyroid glands [10]. In fact, cystic degeneration and hypovascularization are observed after long-term administration of cinacalcet [11].

To destroy hyperplastic parathyroid glands directly, PEIT under ultrasound guidance was developed until cinacalcet became available [7]. However, in addition to injection-related complications such as nerve palsy, ethanol induces severe necrosis in the peri-parathyroid lesion. In addition, repeated injections are needed to control SHPT in some cases [7], which accompanies risks in a series of procedure, and the applications of PEIT are now becoming limited [12].

Etelcalcetide is a novel injectable calcimimetic agent with a mechanism of action similar to that of cinacalcet, and its effect on SHPT is also expected when injected directly into hyperplastic parathyroid glands because it does not induce necrosis in the tissues. The aforementioned past trial required weekly local injection of vitamin D in the parathyroid glands [5]. A previous investigation showed that the terminal half-life of etelcalcetide in HD patients was estimated to be 53 days, excluding HD elimination [6]. Accordingly, we hypothesized that the effect of local etelcalcetide injection would last for a long period of time, such as 8 weeks, because of its pharmacokinetic characteristics.

Calcimimetics represent the most popular treatment for SHPT worldwide, but there are two major drawbacks. First, oral administration of cinacalcet can cause gastrointestinal side effects, such as nausea, which may affect patients' adherence to this drug. However, a newly developed oral calcimimetics, evocalcet, partially overcome the adverse gastrointestinal effects [13]. Second, the cost of calcimimetics in HD therapy is not negligible. If patients are treated with cinacalcet at a dose of 30–60 mg per day, the annual costs will be between \$10,000 and \$19,400 [4], and the cost of calcimimetics accounts for more than 10% of total Medicare dialysis spending [14]. Health insurance in Japan can cover the cost of calcimimetics but may not always be in other countries. Even in Japan, there has been an argument whether the cost of calcimimetics should be bundled in the total HD cost as the same in the USA [14].

In our pilot study, half of the patients achieved an appropriate reduction of iPTH for 8 weeks on average by one local injection of etelcalcetide, resulting in a drastic cost reduction. Systemic administration of etelcalcetide at a dose of 2.5–5 mg per dialysis session costs from \$120 to \$170 a month, whereas the local injection of etelcalcetide given once every 1–2 months costs approximately \$10 for a single treatment. Since our trial included patients who had long-term HD vintage and had taken a large amount of cinacalcet before local injection, further studies including calcimimetics-naïve subjects are warranted.

In conclusion, we performed a direct injection of etelcalcetide in the parathyroid glands safely with drastic cost reduction. Although only half of the patients achieved the target level of iPTH, appropriate selection of subjects may overcome the response rate. Further studies are needed to classify the safety and efficacy of this method. Calcimimetics face the financial pressure of healthcare, but local injection methods of injectable calcimimetics can potentially contribute to the economic aspect of treating SHPT.

References

1. Komaba H. Management of secondary hyperparathyroidism: how and why? Clin Exp Nephrol. 2017;21:37–45.
2. Ketteler M, Block GA, Evenepoel P, Fukagawa M, Herzog CA, McCann L, et al. Executive summary of the 2017 KDIGO Chronic Kidney Disease–Mineral and Bone Disorder (CKD-MBD) guideline update: what's changed and why it matters. Kidney Int. 2017;92:26–36. https://doi.org/10.1016/j.kint.2017.04.006.
3. Tominaga Y, Matsuoka S, Uno N, Sato T. Parathyroidectomy for secondary hyperparathyroidism in the era of calcimimetics. Ther Apher Dial. 2008;12 Suppl. 1.
4. Ziolkowski BS, Abra G. Calcimimetics in end stage renal disease. ASN Kidney News; 2018. https://www.kidneynews.org/kidney-news/features/calcimimetics-in-end-stage-renal-diseas. March: 12.
5. Saito A, Matsumoto Y, Oyama Y, Asaka M, Yokoyama H. Effectiveness of weekly percutaneous maxacalcitol injection therapy in patients with secondary hyperparathyroidism. Ther Apher Dial. 2010;14:98–103.
6. Wu B, Melhem M, Subramanian R, Chen P, Jaramilla Sloey B, Fouqueray B, et al. Clinical pharmacokinetics and pharmacodynamics of etelcalcetide, a novel calcimimetic for treatment of secondary hyperparathyroidism in patients with chronic kidney disease on hemodialysis. J Clin Pharmacol. 2018;58:717–26.
7. Fukugawa M, Kitaoka M, Tominaga Y, Akizawa T, Kakuta T, Onoda N, et al. Guidelines for percutaneous ethanol injection therapy of the parathyroid glands in chronic dialysis patients. Nephrol Dial Transplant. 2003;18(SUPPL. 3):31–3.
8. Funakoshi S, et al. Efficacy of percutaneous etelcalcetide injection into the parathyroid glands on serum parathyroid hormone (PTH) in Hemodialysis (HD) patients with secondary hyperparathyroidism (SHPT): a pilot study. ASN Kidney Week. 2017.
9. Komaba H, Nakanishi S, Fujimori A, Tanaka M, Shin J, Shibuya K, et al. Cinacalcet effectively reduces parathyroid hormone secretion and gland volume regardless of pretreatment gland size in patients with secondary hyperparathyroidism. Clin J Am Soc Nephrol. 2010;5:2305–14.
10. Riccardi D, Martin D. The role of the calcium-sensing receptor in the pathophysiology of secondary hyperparathyroidism. NDT Plus. 2008;1(Suppl 1):7–11.
11. Sumida K, Nakamura M, Ubara Y, Marui Y, Tanaka K, Takaichi K, et al. Histopathological alterations of the parathyroid glands in haemodialysis patients with secondary hyperparathyroidism refractory to cinacalcet hydrochloride. J Clin Pathol. 2011;64:756–60.
12. Meola M, Petrucci I, Barsotti G. Long-term treatment with cinacalcet and conventional therapy reduces parathyroid hyperplasia in severe secondary hyperparathyroidism. Nephrol Dial Transplant. 2009;24:982–9.
13. Kakuta T, Fukagawa M, Kitaoka M, et al. Percutaneous ethanol injection therapy for advanced renal hyperparathyroidism in Japan: 2004 survey by the Japanese Society for Parathyroid Intervention. NDT Plus. 2008;1(Suppl 3):21–5.
14. Fukagawa M, Shimazaki R, Akizawa T. Head-to-head comparison of the new calcimimetic agent evocalcet with cinacalcet in Japanese hemodialysis patients with secondary hyperparathyroidism. Kidney Int. 2018;94:818–25. https://doi.org/10.1016/j.kint.2018.05.013.

Chapter 15
Sudden Cardiac Death in End Stage Kidney Disease: Technologies for Determining Causes and Predicting Risk

Aprajita Mattoo and David M. Charytan

Introduction

As of 2018 there were 785,883 individuals living in the USA with end stage kidney disease (ESKD). A total of 554,038 of these individuals—approximately 70%—were treated for their disease with either peritoneal dialysis (PD) or hemodialysis (HD) [1]. Unfortunately, despite the many advances in renal replacement therapy over the years, the mortality rate for dialysis dependent ESKD patients remains remarkably high. Dialysis patients have an overall mortality that is 10–20 times higher than the general population [1, 2]. The annual mortality rate is approximately 9% per year and the 5-year survival rate for peritoneal dialysis patients and hemodialysis patients are 52% and 42%, respectively [1, 2].

Cardiovascular disease (CVD) is the leading cause of death for individuals on dialysis and accounts for approximately 50% of all known deaths [1, 3, 4]. Sudden cardiac death (SCD) accounts for the majority of all CVD deaths in dialysis patients and occurs at a rate almost 20 times greater than that of the general population. Extensive research in this area has shown that the association of SCD and HD patients is independent of traditional CVD risk factors and coronary artery disease severity, and strongly suggest unique causes for SCD in the HD population [5, 6]. Mechanisms proposed for the prevalence of SCD in dialysis patients include chronic inflammation, endothelial dysfunction, vascular calcification, myocardial hypertrophy, and uremic cardiomyopathy [7]. More recently, a number of studies have focused on investigating and describing the different cardiac arrhythmias and electrolyte derangements underlying SCD events in HD patients. In this review we will

A. Mattoo · D. M. Charytan (✉)
Nephrology Division, NYU Grossman School of Medicine, New York, NY, USA
e-mail: Aprajita.Mattoo@nyulangone.org; david.charytan@nyulangone.org

S. J. Saggi, M. O. Salifu (eds.), *Technological Advances in Care of Patients with Kidney Diseases*, https://doi.org/10.1007/978-3-031-11942-2_15

discuss these cardiac arrythmias and electrolyte abnormalities implicated in SCD in HD patients as well as contemporary technologies that may be utilized to identify these pathologies and predict the risk of SCD.

Cardiac Arrythmias and Sudden Cardiac Death in ESKD

Over the past 50 years there has been substantial literature describing the relationship between cardiac arrhythmias and SCD in HD patients [8]. Thanks to advances in continuous cardiac monitoring, our understanding of what types of underlying arrhythmias can lead to SCD in this population has evolved. Early studies emphasized the role of ventricular arrhythmias in SCD, while more recent research suggests that atrial and brady arrythmias play an important part as well [8]. A complexity of this research, however, lies in the basic definition of SCD. SCD is defined as an unexpected death due to cardiac causes in a person with known or unknown cardiac disease, within 1 h of symptom onset (witnessed SCD) or within 24 h of the last proof of life (unwitnessed SCD). Given this broad definition, SCD is subject to misclassification in research studies. As such, while SCD is a leading cause of death in HD patients, it is important to recognize the uncertainty around estimated rates of SCD engendered by this definition or reliance on categorization of unexpected deaths as SCD by the treating clinical providers (e.g., on the United States Renal Data System Death Notification Form) and the likely inclusion of both SCD definitively due to sudden cardiac arrest (SCA), deaths due to other adverse cerebral and CV events, and non-cardiovascular sudden deaths such those due to drug overdose.

Ventricular Arrythmia

Initial studies in SCD in HD patients utilized 12-lead electrocardiograms (ECG) and ambulatory ECG recording systems (such as Holter monitors and wearable cardioverter-defibrillators) to investigate the types of terminal cardiac arrythmias that preceded a cardiac event or death. These initial studies suggested ventricular arrythmia as the predominant terminal arrythmia in SCD in HD patients. In retrospect, however, these initial studies had several limitations. The Gruppo Emodialisi e Patologie Cardiovasculari studied 127 HD patients using 48-h Holter monitoring and found the incidence of ventricular arrhythmia to be 76% [9]. Ventricular arrythmias in this study, however, were defined as greater than or equal to two PVCs in an hour and were classified by the Lown PVC Scoring System; a classification of 4A represented PVC couplets and a classification of 4B represented greater than or equal to three PVCs (i.e., ventricular tachycardia) [9]. Twenty nine percent of patients had greater than or equal to two PVCs in a hour, 21% of patients had Lown's 4A or 4B findings, and 6% of patients had ventricular tachycardia. The study did not evaluate mortality and only one patient died of SCD out of the 127 enrolled [9].

A study by Bozbas et al. involving 94 HD patients who underwent 24-h Holter monitoring showed the incidence ventricular arrythmia to be 85.1%, with 37.2% of cases being classified as complex ventricular arrhythmias [10]. In this study ventricular arrythmia was also classified by the Lown PVC Scoring System with a classification of 3 (i.e., multiform PVCs) and above being defined as complex ventricular arrythmias [10]. Similar to the Gruppo Emodialisi e Patologie Cardiovasculari study, the association of these complex ventricular arrythmias with SCD or mortality was not specifically addressed [10]. Davis et al. on the other hand looked at 110 HD patients who experienced SCD in outpatient dialysis facilities over a 14-year period. Initial ECG rhythms performed at the time of SCD showed that ventricular fibrillation and ventricular tachycardia accounted for 67% of cases while pulseless electrical activity and asystole accounted for only 33% [11]. Interestingly, in this study the 1-year mortality of VF/VT cases was higher than PEA/asystole cases (81% vs. 95%) [11]. A clear limitation of this study is that inclusion required performance of an ECG at the time of a witnessed arrest making generalizability of the findings to the majority of patients with unwitnessed arrest uncertain [11]. Ultimately, the most persuasive study addressing the relationship between by ventricular arrythmias and SCD was a study by Wan et al. [12]. This group studied 75 HD patients who had survived a prior arrest and evaluated the relationship between ventricular arrhythmia, SCD, and survival [12]. They described 84 SCA events (119 arrhythmia episodes) while wearing a wearable cardioverter-defibrillators and found that that 78.6% of SCAs were due to ventricular tachycardia or ventricular fibrillation and 21.4% were due to asystole [12]. They also found acute 24-h survival to be 70.7% for all SCA events; 30-day and 1-year survival were 50.7% and 31.4%, respectively [12].

Atrial Fibrillation

Atrial fibrillation (AF) has been shown to be an independent risk factor for SCD in numerous studies performed in cardiac patients and the general population [13]. While the exact mechanism of death is not fully understood, a fast ventricular rate in the context of atrial tachycardia can reduce ventricular refractoriness and promote the occurrence of lethal ventricular arrhythmias and subsequent SCD [8]. Research over the past 15 years has resulted in AF being increasingly recognized as a prevailing arrythmia in HD patients [14, 15], though no study to date has shown a direct pathologic link between atrial fibrillation and SCD. Goldstein et al. studied 258,605 HD patients and found the incidence rate of AF to be 14.8/100 person-years [14]. In their study of 256 patients on long-term HD, Vazquez et al. demonstrated both a high prevalence of AF (12.1%) as well as significance as an independent risk factor for 1.7-fold increase in mortality [16]. Unfortunately this study also did not evaluate for a relationship between atrial fibrillation and SCD [16]. Genovesi et al. evaluated 488 patients on long-term HD and found the prevalence of atrial fibrillation to be 27%, a prevalence 3–15 times greater than in the Framingham population according to age groups [17]. Subsequent studies by Genovesi et al. on 476 long-term HD patients found that AF was independently associated with increased cardiovascular mortality, increased overall mortality, and SCD [18, 19].

Bradycardia

Perhaps the most interesting research on the relationship between cardiac arrhythmia and SCD has emerged in the past 5 years from studies utilizing implantable loop recorders (ILR) on HD dependent ESKD populations [20]. These studies represent the most compelling data thus far regarding the nature of malignant cardiac rhythms in HD patients, and they have all suggested that brady-arrythmias have an important role in the development of in SCD [21–25]. Roy-Chaudhury et al. used ILRs to continuously monitor heart rhythms for approximately 6 months in 66 ESKD patients on HD. His group found that bradycardias and asystole accounted for a much higher proportion of serious arrythmias than ventricular tachycardia. Out of 1678 clinically significant events recorded by ILRs, 1461 events were bradycardias, with 14 episodes of asystole and only one episode of sustained ventricular tachycardia [22]. There were no cases of SCD noted in the study. Sacher et al. studied 71 HD patients for approximately 21 months and identified a greater incidence rate of combined brady arrhythmias and asystole than for ventricular arrhythmias (14/100 patient-years versus 9/100 patient-years, respectively) [23]. Moreover, the terminal rhythm in the four patients with SCD was progressive bradycardia followed by asystole [23]. There were no instances of primary ventricular arrythmia leading to SCD in their study [23]. Wong et al. followed 50 ESKD patients on HD with ILRs for approximately 18 months and found that out of a total of 1586 clinically significant events recorded by ILRs, 30% of events were bradycardia, 28% were asystole/sinus arrest, 8% were second-degree AV block, and only 20% were ventricular tachycardia [24]. More importantly, SCD occurred in 16% of patients, and for each recorded case the terminal event captured was severe bradycardia and asystole. No episodes of ventricular tachycardia associated with SCD were detected [24]. Additional studies using ILRs to evaluate SCD in HD patients have yielded similar results, supporting the perspective that while ventricular arrythmias are a common finding among HD patients, bradyarrhythmia's are likely to play a more important role when it comes to SCD [25, 26].

Electrolyte Abnormalities and Sudden Cardic Death in ESKD

An association between pre-dialytic serum electrolyte value or the dialysate electrolyte concentration and the risk of sudden death is well established.

Potassium and SCD

Pre-dialytic hyperkalemia and hypokalemia have both been shown to increase mortality and the risk of SCD in ESKD patients on HD. Sacher et al. showed that the risk of cardiac conduction disorders increased with serum potassium concentrations >5.0 mmol/L and that ventricular arrhythmias increased with serum plasma potassium concentrations <4.0 mmol/L [23]. Kovesdy et al. demonstrated in a study involving 81,013 HD patients that were followed for approximately 3 years that a potassium concentrations between 4.6 and 5.3 mEq/L were associated with the greatest survival and that both a "high" serum potassium of >5.6 mEq/L and a "low" serum potassium of <4.0 mEq/L were associated with increased mortality [27]. Similarly, Pun et al. studied 2134 patients on HD and found the incidence rate of SCA to be 4.5/100,000 dialysis treatments: a pre-dialysis serum potassium level of 5.1 mEq/L was associated with the lowest risk of peri-dialytic sudden cardiac arrest, whereas potassium levels above and below 5.1 were associated with increasing risk for SCD [28]. Genovesi et al. studied 476 long-term HD patients and found SCD had a 6.9% cumulative incidence, and that pre-dialytic hyperkalemia was a significant predictor of SCD [19]. The importance of pre-dialysis serum hyperkalemia is also suggested by the increased incidence of cardiovascular deaths and CV hospitalizations noted on the first days of the dialytic week, when the severity of hyperkalemia is most marked [20, 29].

In addition to the ramifications of pre-dialytic potassium levels on SCD, the potassium concentrations of the dialysate used in HD sessions have also been shown to increase the risk for SCD. Three large cohort observational studies have described associations between low-potassium dialysate (<2 mEq/L) and SCD in outpatient dialysis units. Pun et al. studied 2134 patients on HD and found that patients who experienced SCD were significantly more likely to be exposed to low potassium dialysate (less than 2 mEq/L) during their last recorded HD session as compared to HD patients who did not experience SCD (17.7% vs. 9.3%) [28]. Similarly, a study by Karnik et al. that evaluated 400 cases of SCD in patients on HD found that patients with SCD were nearly twice as likely to have been dialyzed against a low potassium (0 or 1.0 mEq/L) dialysate on the day of cardiac arrest (17.1% vs. 8.8%) as opposed to patients who did not have SCD [30]. Finally, a study by Jadoul et al. evaluated 37,765 patients on HD and found an association between low potassium dialysate (<1.5 mEq/L and <2–2.5 mEq/L) and SCD [31].

Calcium and SCD

Serum and dialysate calcium levels have also been associated with an increased risk mortality and SCD in HD patients [32]. Epidemiologic data shows that both low and high serum pre-dialysis calcium levels are associated with higher mortality in HD patients. In a study of 107,200 HD patients by Miller et al. both lower and higher pre-dialysis serum calcium levels (<9.0 and >10.0 mg/dL, respectively) were associated with higher mortality risk [32].

Analyses of the dialysate calcium concentration have had mixed results. In a study of 2134 HD patients, Pun et al. found that dialysate calcium concentrations <2.5 mEq/L were associated with higher risk of SCD [28]. In a subsequent study, this group evaluated 510 HD patients who experienced SCD and found that a higher serum Ca, a low Ca dialysate (<2.5 mEq/L), and an increasing serum dialysate Ca gradient were associated with an increased risk of SCD. Exposure to low calcium dialysate (<2.5 mEq/L) was associated with a dramatic, 40% increase in the risk of SCD [33]. However, a secondary analysis of 3883 hemodialysis patients from the EVOLVE trial did not observe an association between dialysate calcium concentrations (categorized as <2.5, 2.5, vs. ≥2.5 meq/L) and cardiovascular death or SCD [34]. These conflicting findings demonstrate the need for more research in the area of calcium homeostasis and SCD [34].

Bicarbonate and SCD

Studies examining the relationship between bicarbonate level, mortality, and SCD have had varying conclusions. Both high and low pre-dialysis serum bicarbonate levels have been associated with an increased risk of mortality in studies of patients receiving HD [35]. Wu et al. studied 56,835 HD patients and showed that low pre-dialysis serum bicarbonate level (serum bicarbonate <22 mEq/L) was associated with a higher risk of death [36]. Conversely, Bommer et al. evaluated 7000 patients on HD and found that both low (≤17 mEq/L) and high (>27 mEq/L) pre-dialysis serum bicarbonate levels were associated with an increased risk for mortality [37]. Studies have also examined associations with dialysate bicarbonate concentration. Tentori et al. evaluated 17,031 HD patients and found that there was a trend towards higher risks of all-cause mortality and SCD with higher dialysate bicarbonate concentrations [38].

Although these data are compelling, it is important to mention that the cumulative literature on serum electrolyte abnormalities, dialysate composition, mortality, and SCD have failed to distinguish between the extent to which risk is related to the absolute value of the plasma or dialysate electrolyte value, versus the extent to which intradialytic electrolyte shifts across concentration gradients during HD contribute to a pro-arrhythmogenic milieu for SCD. Shifts can persist after the HD session is completed and are thought to be one of the reasons why there is a high risk of SCD in the hours following HD sessions [39].

Utilizing current and emerging technologies to both define the underlying cardiac arrhythmia and predict the likelihood of a cardiovascular event holds great promise for preventing cardiac arrhythmias that may lead to SCD, but has thus far not been tested.

Approaches to Defining the Underlying Cardiac Arrythmias in SCD AND ESKD

Implantable Loop Recorders

Early studies concerning cardiac arrythmias and SCD in ESKD were typically performed with 12 lead ECG, Holter monitors, or wearable cardioverter-defibrillators. While these technologies were accurate, their relatively short duration of cardiac monitoring capability limited the ability to reliably capture dialysis associated arrythmia and SCD events. As briefly noted above, several recent studies have utilized implantable loop recorders (ILRs) to better understand the underlying cardiac rhythms associated with SCD in ESRD. ILR are minimally invasive and can be inserted subcutaneously under local anesthesia during a brief procedure. They allow for continuous cardiac monitoring from several weeks to several years. In the past 5 years there have been five major studies using ILRs in HD patients that have significantly impacted the current understanding of the terminal arrythmias associated with SCD and ESKD. Silva et al. [25], Roy Chaudhury et al. [22], Sacher et al. [23], Roberts et al. [26], and Wong et al. [24] all performed studies evaluating SCD in HD patients using ILRs. The results of these studies have highlighted the role brady arrhythmias may play in the development of SCD and shifted the emphasis away from ventricular arrythmias [21]. All-cause mortality was similar across the studies (0.14 deaths per patient year of follow-up) and the incidence of SCD was 0.06. Although there was some variation in rates across the studies, 40% of deaths were classified as SCD [21]. ILRs revealed that brady arrhythmias/asystole were more common than VT/VF (combined annualized rate of brady arrythmias/asystole was 0.19 versus a combined annualized rate for VT/VF of 0.02) [21].

ILR studies have also yielded important results regarding the timing of SCD in HD patients. For example, Roy-Chaudhury et al. [22] demonstrated that the pattern of detected arrhythmias closely mimicked the temporal pattern of CV events and SCD with dramatic spikes in arrhythmia frequency occurring during the first HD session of the week when electrolyte flux is maximal.

ECG Patch Monitors

Although ILR represented a significant advancement compared with 12-lead ECG machines, Holter monitors, event monitors or wearable cardioverter-defibrillators, the requirement for a (minimally) invasive implant procedure limits their use and acceptability. Recent advances in ECG technology, however, have led to the development of new "patch" ECG devices that are compact, wireless, energy efficient, and capable of an extended duration of continuous cardiac monitoring. These devices usually consist of an adhesive patch, a sensor, a microelectronic circuit with recorder and memory storage, and an internal battery embedded in a relatively flexible matrix or resin. The Zio XT Patch (iRhythm Technologies Inc., San Francisco, CA, USA) is an example of such a device. It is a single channel patch ECG that can provide up to 2 weeks of continuous cardiac monitoring. It is medical grade device, FDA approved, and has been clinically validated in several cardiovascular studies. The ability to perform continuous ECG monitoring for both symptomatic and asymptomatic cardiac arrythmias in patients prior to, during, and following HD could provide a wealth of diagnostic information relating to cardiac arrythmias and the incidence of SCD in ESKD. Rogovoy et al. utilized a "patch" ECG monitor in such a way. This group used a Zio XT Patch to perform continuous ECG monitoring for 14 days on a cohort of 28 ESKD patients and found that 46% of patients experienced arrythmias. Non-sustained VT was more frequent during dialysis or within 6 h post-dialysis as compared to pre-dialysis (63% vs 37%). Supraventricular tachycardia was more frequent pre dialysis as compared to during dialysis or within 6 h post dialysis (84% vs. 16%) [40].

Implantable Cardioverter Defibrillators

Implantable cardioverter-defibrillators (ICD) are more invasive than ILR or ECG "patch" monitors and are generally inserted for therapeutic rather than diagnostic purposes. However, they have also been used for long-term cardiac monitoring in dialysis patients. The Implantable Cardioverter Defibrillator-2 Trial (ICD2) was a prospective, randomized controlled study of primary prevention ICD therapy in dialysis patients [41]. While the study was principally designed to evaluate the effectiveness of ICDs in preventing SCD in ESKD as reviewed below, it revealed significant information regarding the types of cardiac arrhythmias associated with hemodialysis. An analysis of cardiac arrhythmia among participants found that AF was present in 14 of 40 dialysis patients and clearly correlated with the dialysis cycle with a threefold higher incidence on dialysis days and a 13-fold higher incidence during HD than in the 7 h before dialysis [42].

Approaches to Predicting the Risk of Sudden Death

Autonomic Tone and Sudden Cardiac Death

Abnormalities in autonomic tone, particularly sympathetic drive, have been associated with SCD in the general population, the CVD population, and the ESKD population. Indeed, the high sympathetic output in ESKD patients is supported by an association between high circulating levels of norepinephrine in this patient population and cardiac events, such as SCD [43]. One measure of autonomic tone and sympathetic drive is heart rate variability (HRV), which identifies the variation in successive heart beats (the inter-beat interval, also known as the R-R interval) either by time-domain or frequency-domain measurements. Several studies have suggested that measuring HRV is a potential method of risk stratification of HD patients for risk of SCD. For example, Oikawa et al. assessed HRV in 383 long-term HD patients and found that decreased HRV was an independent predictor of all-cause mortality and cardiovascular mortality, including SCD [44]. Nishimura et al. studied 196 HD patients and found that a low frequency HRV to high frequency HRV ratio (LF/HF) of >1.9 was associated with an increased risk of SCD; at 5 years only 29.4% of patients with a LF/HF ratio greater than 1.9 remained free of SCD [45].

Research into HRV and other measures of autonomic tone in HD patients has always been limited by the difficulty of performing continuous monitoring studies prior to, during, and following HD. The rise in smart, wearable technologies in the past decade however has prompted a renewed interest in better understanding the relationship of HRV and SCD in HD patients. Smart, wearable technologies include medical grade devices as well as commercially available consumer products. The Bittium Faros TM 360 (Bittium Corporation, Oulu, Finland) and the Actiheart 5 (CamNtech Ltd., Cambridgeshire, United Kingdom) are patch ECGs that are capable of measuring HRV. FitBit, Apple, and Omron watches are consumer products with the ability to report on heart rate, blood oximetry, cardiac monitoring, and blood pressure. While the ability to report on HRV, is currently crude, this is anticipated to improve in the future, although sophisticated algorithms will be needed to reliably report HRV in the setting of the frequent premature ventricular and atrial contractions that occur in the setting of ESKD. Furthermore, calculation of HRV may not be feasible in the setting of AF which is common in this population. On the other hand, several of these products are FDA-approved and there is a growing body of literature in neurology, sleep, psychiatry, and cardiovascular disease looking to validate their clinical applications for a whole host of conditions including seizure, obstructive sleep apnea, schizophrenia, heart failure, and sudden cardiac death.

Electrophysiology and Sudden Cardiac Death

Early studies looking at the role of 12-lead ECG in predicting SCD in HD patients focused on the QT interval (or heart rate corrected interval, QTc). The QTc interval reflects the total duration of ventricular depolarization and re-polarization. Since ventricular depolarization is usually fixed (as reflected by QRS duration), short-term variations in QTc interval primarily reflect variations in ventricular re-polarization. The QTc interval can be affected by a variety of parameters including electrolyte shifts, acidosis, medications, changes in autonomic tone, cardiac disease, and left ventricular hypertrophy [46]. Thus, it is difficult to fully elucidate a direct cause-and-effect relationship between QTc interval and SCD. Regardless, a prolonged QTc interval has long been associated with SCD and ventricular arrhythmias in various populations, including dialysis patients [46]. In a study by Genovesi et al., the QTc interval was evaluated in 122 patients on chronic hemodialysis [47]. A prolonged QTc was present in 36% of patients and was associated with increased total mortality and an even higher increased risk of SCD [47]. Moreover, in a subgroup of 44 patients with very prolonged QTc intervals (≥480 ms), 29.5% of patients died, and 46% of those deaths were attributed to SCD [47]. Similarly, Hage et al. evaluated 280 patients with ESKD and found that a longer QTc interval was associated with increased total mortality even after adjusting for factors such as LVH, LVEF, and CAD severity [48]. Unfortunately, while these studies all demonstrate an association of QTc prolongation and SCD in dialysis patients, it remains unclear if the relationship is truly related to SCD and arrhythmia or if it is reflective of concomitant conditions such as electrolyte derangements, cardiac disease, and left ventricular hypertrophy [46]. Nevertheless, these studies do suggest that a obtaining a routine EKG has significant potential to predict SCD risk in the dialysis population, although it may not help to identify the underlying etiology of increased risk at this time.

Recently there has been interest in using advanced computerized analysis of ECGs to better understand the relationship between HD and SCD. The spatial QRS-T angle is an established marker of global cardiac depolarization and repolarization that can be measured from a standard 12 lead ECG. A wide spatial QRS-T angle has been associated with total mortality and SCD in several populations, including HD patients [46, 49]. De Bie et al. evaluated 277 HD patients and found that the spatial QRS-T angle was abnormal in 35% of patients and was associated with a significant increase in the risk of all-cause mortality and SCD [50]. However, an abnormal spatial QRS-T angle in this study was more frequent in those with CAD, diabetes, LVH, reduced LVEF, and longer QTc intervals, thus muddling the nature of the association between spatial QRS-T angle and SCD in HD patients. Another study by Tereshchenko et al. of a cohort of 358 HD patients showed that a spatial QRS-T angle >75% was associated with all-cause mortality, CV mortality, and SCD [51]. However, the authors noted that while spatial QRS-T angle shows promise as a non-invasive test for SCD risk stratification, additional studies are required to understand the optimal abnormal cut off value for spatial QRS-T angle in the HD population.

Positron Emission Tomography and Sudden Cardiac Death

Positron emission tomography (PET) is another, emerging technology to predict SCD risk in HD patients. Global coronary flow reserve (CFR) assessed by PET is a noninvasive, quantitative indicator of myocardial perfusion and ischemia that integrates the hemodynamic effects of epicardial stenosis, diffuse atherosclerosis, and microvascular dysfunction [52]. CFR/PET has been studied in several cohorts at high risk for cardiovascular death [52, 53] and has been shown to improve the value of traditional risk assessments [i.e., Duke Clinical Risk Score, Rest left ventricular ejection fraction (LVEF), LVEF reserve, etc.] and to be an independent correlate of cardiovascular and all-cause mortality. Given this data, Shah et al. retrospectively evaluated the prognostic value of CFR/PET in 168 HD patients who underwent rest and stress myocardial perfusion PET, and they found that global CFR was independently associated with cardiovascular mortality and all-cause mortality [52]. For all-cause mortality, the addition of global CFR/PET resulted in risk reclassification in 27% of patients. Thus, global CFR provided independent and incremental risk stratification for all-cause and cardiovascular mortality in patients with ESKD and as such may provide useful technology for SCD risk stratification [52].

Implantable Cardioverter Defibrillators and Sudden Cardiac Death

Several important clinical trials have demonstrated that implantable cardioverter-defibrillators (ICDs) offer a significant survival benefit in high-risk patients for either primary or secondary prevention of sudden cardiac death. These high-risk patient populations included cardiovascular patients with reduced systolic left ventricular function or those with a history of ventricular arrythmia. Patients on HD, despite their high incidence of SCD, were not included in these studies. As such the role of ICDs for either primary or secondary prevention of SCD in ESKD is less clear.

Observational studies have also looked at the role of ICDs in HD patients in order to better understand the possibility of benefit from ICD therapy. Pun et al. analyzed 108 patients on HD in the US National Cardiovascular Data Registry's ICD Registry who had undergone ICD placement for primary prevention and compared them to 195 patients with low ejection fraction but without an ICD from the Get With the Guidelines-Heart Failure database. In HD patients with a primary prevention ICD, 1- and 3-year mortality rates were 42.2% and 68.8%, respectively. In patients without ICDs, the 1- and 3-year mortality rates were comparable at 38.1% and 75.7%, respectively. Thus ICD use for primary prevention in HD patients was not associated with a significant survival advantage [54]. Another large study by Charytan et al. retrospectively reviewed 9528 HD patients who received either primary or secondary prevention ICD and found that the incidence of death after ICD implantation was high, with 448 deaths/1000 patient-years, predominantly due to cardiovascular events [55]. The risk of infection was even greater, at 515 events/1000 patient-years. Importantly, among HD patients who were given an ICD for secondary prevention there was a significant survival advantage associated with ICD implantation when compared with a control group, although that benefit was attenuated after 3 years [55].

The Implantable Cardioverter-Defibrillator in Dialysis Patients (ICD2) Study was the first RCT to explore the efficacy of prophylactic ICD implantation in dialysis patients. Ninety-seven HD patients were randomized to ICD placement and 91 to the control group over an enrollment period of 12 years [56]. The trial was stopped early for futility at the recommendation of the data safety and monitoring group. During a median follow up period of 6.8 years, SCD occurred in 7.9% of ICD patients and 9.7% of the control group. The 5-year probability of survival was 50.6% in the ICD group and 54.5% in the control group. Additionally, 7.5% of ICD patients enrolled required explanation of the device, mostly due to infection. The study authors concluded that in a well screened and treated HD population, prophylactic ICD therapy did not reduce SCD or all-cause mortality. On the basis of these studies, ICD implantation cannot be routinely recommended for primary prevention of SCD in ESKD patients on chronic HD at this time, although questions remain regarding the appropriate role in secondary prevention.

Electrophysiology and Point of Care and Sudden Cardiac Death

Monitoring changes in electrolyte concentrations around a patient's HD session presents an interesting approach to SCD risk stratification in the setting of ESKD. ECG cardiac monitoring is one potential approach as ECG morphology can reflect changes in electrolyte concentrations. For example, peaked T-waves, U waves, and QT interval changes have been classically used to diagnose, hyperkalemia, hypokalemia, hypocalcemia, and hypercalcemia. Utilizing ECG morphology to track electrolyte changes around HD has not yet been attempted in any major study, but it should become more feasible as ECG patch technology continues to evolve. In addition to ECG monitoring, several new point of care devices would also allow for monitoring of electrolytes around a patient's HD session. The iSTAT System (fully portable) and the Piccolo Xpress (Abbot Point of Care, Princeton, New Jersey, USA) are small, blood analyzer devices that yield reliable test results in 2 min and 12 min of sample procurement, respectively. These devices have been used in a variety of settings requiring rapid turnaround time (for example, troponin testing in emergency rooms) with excellent results. ECG monitoring to assess electrolyte levels or measurement with point of care chemistry devices might allow monitoring of electrolyte concentration prior to dialysis as well as the dynamic peridialytic changes. Although not yet tested, their use could facilitate a move away from the current standard practice of adjusting the dialysis prescription on the basis of once monthly labs in favor of altering the prescription at each HD session or with real-time, intradialytic adjustment of the HD prescription in response to the detection of out-of-range changes in electrolytes during an HD session. In theory, this type of approach could limit the occurrence of hyperkalemia, hypokalemia and other electrolyte abnormalities that predispose to the occurrence of SCD.

Artificial Intelligence and Sudden Cardiac Death

Artificial intelligence and machine learning (AI/ML) solutions are present in almost every field of medicine and are likely to have increasing role to play in the ESKD population. While no study to date has evaluated the role of these tools for predicting SCD in HD patients, studies have been performed that predict cardiovascular outcomes, intradialytic hemodynamic events, mortality and survival in HD patients [57]. For example, Akbilgic et al. conducted a study using machine learning to help predict mortality after HD initiation. Using data from electronic health records (EHR) on a cohort of 27,615 ESKD patients, they created an algorithm that could predict outcomes on 30-, 90-, 180-, and 365-day all-cause mortality after dialysis initiation. The model showed good internal validity and replicated well in patients with various demographic and clinical characteristics [58]. Similar AI/ML models could be created in the future to predict HD at high risk of SCD utilizing big data from ESKD registries, EHR, and cardiovascular studies. Moreover, advancements in AI have also led to the integration of machine learning and deep learning technologies in many medical devices. For example, machine learning algorithms based off of Zio XT ECG patch data has helped to create a new generation of Zio XT devices with greater diagnostic accuracy [59]. KardiaMobile (AliveCor Inc., San Francisco, CA, USA) is another single channel patch ECG that is a medical grade, FDA-approved device that works with smartphone technology to allow for real time monitoring and recording of cardiac rhythms for up to 200 h. It has been utilized in studies involving deep learning AI to help with the detection of hyperkalemia. Galloway et al. utilized a deep neural network trained to detect hyperkalemia by ECG morphology as detected by AliveCor smartphone device [60]. Subsequently, the same device was used to record ECGs during dialysis sessions, with concurrent blood testing. Potassium was predicted with an error of only 9% suggesting that the device and algorithm was a viable tool for detecting hyperkalemia [61]. In combination with a smartphone ECG, this machine learning approach may enable a new means for rapid, non-invasive monitoring and screening for hyperkalemia during HD and allow for real time HD prescription adjustments to be made to avoid SCD [57]. Thus AI/ML offers the potential for a big data approach to identify HD patients at high risk of SCD as well the potential of a personalized medicine approach to HD prescription management to reduce the risk of SCD.

Conclusion

SCD remains a leading cause of death in ESKD patients. Significant research has been performed to better understand the precipitants of SCD. Emerging technologies offer exciting opportunities to better identify and stratify high risk ESKD patients.

References

1. https://adr.usrds.org/2020/end-stage-renal-disease/5-mortality.
2. Mavrakanas TA, Charytan DM. Cardiovascular complications in chronic dialysis patients. Curr Opin Nephrol Hypertens. 2016;25(6):536–44. https://doi.org/10.1097/MNH.0000000000000280.
3. Sarnak MJ, Amann K, Bangalore S, et al. Chronic kidney disease and coronary artery disease: JACC state-of-the-art review. J Am Coll Cardiol. 2019;74(14):1823–38. https://doi.org/10.1016/j.jacc.2019.08.1017.
4. Boyle NG, Do DH. Hemodialysis patients: high risk for sudden death, but what is the cause? JACC Clin Electrophysiol. 2018;4(3):409–11. https://doi.org/10.1016/j.jacep.2017.09.005.
5. Makar MS, Pun PH. Sudden cardiac death among hemodialysis patients. Am J Kidney Dis. 2017;69(5):684–95. https://doi.org/10.1053/j.ajkd.2016.12.006.
6. Pun PH, Smarz TR, Honeycutt EF, Shaw LK, Al-Khatib SM, Middleton JP. Chronic kidney disease is associated with increased risk of sudden cardiac death among patients with coronary artery disease. Kidney Int. 2009;76(6):652–8. https://doi.org/10.1038/ki.2009.219.
7. Himmelfarb J, Stenvinkel P, Ikizler TA, Hakim RM. The elephant in uremia: oxidant stress as a unifying concept of cardiovascular disease in uremia. Kidney Int. 2002;62(5):1524–38. https://doi.org/10.1046/j.1523-1755.2002.00600.x.
8. Samanta R, Chan C, Chauhan VS. Arrhythmias and sudden cardiac death in end stage renal disease: epidemiology, risk factors, and management. Can J Cardiol. 2019;35(9):1228–40. https://doi.org/10.1016/j.cjca.2019.05.005.
9. Multicentre, cross-sectional study of ventricular arrhythmias in chronically haemodialysed patients. Gruppo Emodialisi e Patologie Cardiovasculari. Lancet. 1988;2(8606):305–9. https://www.ncbi.nlm.nih.gov/pubmed/2899721.
10. Bozbas H, Atar I, Yildirir A, et al. Prevalence and predictors of arrhythmia in end stage renal disease patients on hemodialysis. Ren Fail. 2007;29(3):331–9. https://doi.org/10.1080/08860220701191237.
11. Davis TR, Young BA, Eisenberg MS, Rea TD, Copass MK, Cobb LA. Outcome of cardiac arrests attended by emergency medical services staff at community outpatient dialysis centers. Kidney Int. 2008;73(8):933–9. https://doi.org/10.1038/sj.ki.5002749.
12. Wan C, Herzog CA, Zareba W, Szymkiewicz SJ. Sudden cardiac arrest in hemodialysis patients with wearable cardioverter defibrillator. Ann Noninvasive Electrocardiol. 2014;19(3):247–57. https://doi.org/10.1111/anec.12119.
13. Eisen A, Ruff CT, Braunwald E, et al. Sudden cardiac death in patients with atrial fibrillation: insights from the ENGAGE AF-TIMI 48 trial. J Am Heart Assoc. 2016;5(7):e003735. https://doi.org/10.1161/JAHA.116.003735.
14. Goldstein BA, Arce CM, Hlatky MA, Turakhia M, Setoguchi S, Winkelmayer WC. Trends in the incidence of atrial fibrillation in older patients initiating dialysis in the United States. Circulation. 2012;126(19):2293–301. https://doi.org/10.1161/CIRCULATIONAHA.112.099606.
15. Winkelmayer WC, Patrick AR, Liu J, Brookhart MA, Setoguchi S. The increasing prevalence of atrial fibrillation among hemodialysis patients. J Am Soc Nephrol. 2011;22(2):349–57. https://doi.org/10.1681/ASN.2010050459.
16. Vazquez E, Sanchez-Perales C, Garcia-Garcia F, et al. Atrial fibrillation in incident dialysis patients. Kidney Int. 2009;76(3):324–30. https://doi.org/10.1038/ki.2009.185.
17. Genovesi S, Pogliani D, Faini A, et al. Prevalence of atrial fibrillation and associated factors in a population of long-term hemodialysis patients. Am J Kidney Dis. 2005;46(5):897–902. https://doi.org/10.1053/j.ajkd.2005.07.044.
18. Genovesi S, Vincenti A, Rossi E, et al. Atrial fibrillation and morbidity and mortality in a cohort of long-term hemodialysis patients. Am J Kidney Dis. 2008;51(2):255–62. https://doi.org/10.1053/j.ajkd.2007.10.034.

19. Genovesi S, Valsecchi MG, Rossi E, et al. Sudden death and associated factors in a historical cohort of chronic haemodialysis patients. Nephrol Dial Transplant. 2009;24(8):2529–36. https://doi.org/10.1093/ndt/gfp104.
20. Charytan DM, Foley R, McCullough PA, et al. Arrhythmia and sudden death in hemodialysis patients: protocol and baseline characteristics of the monitoring in dialysis study. Clin J Am Soc Nephrol. 2016;11(4):721–34. https://doi.org/10.2215/CJN.09350915.
21. Roberts PR, Stromberg K, Johnson LC, Wiles BM, Mavrakanas TA, Charytan DM. A systematic review of the incidence of arrhythmias in hemodialysis patients undergoing long-term monitoring with implantable loop recorders. Kidney Int Rep. 2021;6(1):56–65. https://doi.org/10.1016/j.ekir.2020.10.020.
22. Roy-Chaudhury P, Tumlin JA, Koplan BA, et al. Primary outcomes of the Monitoring in Dialysis Study indicate that clinically significant arrhythmias are common in hemodialysis patients and related to dialytic cycle. Kidney Int. 2018;93(4):941–51. https://doi.org/10.1016/j.kint.2017.11.019.
23. Sacher F, Jesel L, Borni-Duval C, et al. Cardiac rhythm disturbances in hemodialysis patients: early detection using an implantable loop recorder and correlation with biological and dialysis parameters. JACC Clin Electrophysiol. 2018;4(3):397–408. https://doi.org/10.1016/j.jacep.2017.08.002.
24. Wong MCG, Kalman JM, Pedagogos E, et al. Bradycardia and asystole is the predominant mechanism of sudden cardiac death in patients with chronic kidney disease. J Am Coll Cardiol. 2015;65(12):1263–5. https://doi.org/10.1016/j.jacc.2014.12.049.
25. Silva RT, Martinelli Filho M, Peixoto Gde L, et al. Predictors of arrhythmic events detected by implantable loop recorders in renal transplant candidates. Arq Bras Cardiol. 2015;105(5):493–502. https://doi.org/10.5935/abc.20150106.
26. Roberts PR, Zachariah D, Morgan JM, et al. Monitoring of arrhythmia and sudden death in a hemodialysis population: the CRASH-ILR study. PLoS One. 2017;12(12):e0188713. https://doi.org/10.1371/journal.pone.0188713.
27. Kovesdy CP, Regidor DL, Mehrotra R, et al. Serum and dialysate potassium concentrations and survival in hemodialysis patients. Clin J Am Soc Nephrol. 2007;2(5):999–1007. https://doi.org/10.2215/CJN.04451206.
28. Pun PH, Lehrich RW, Honeycutt EF, Herzog CA, Middleton JP. Modifiable risk factors associated with sudden cardiac arrest within hemodialysis clinics. Kidney Int. 2011;79(2):218–27. https://doi.org/10.1038/ki.2010.315.
29. Foley RN, Gilbertson DT, Murray T, Collins AJ. Long interdialytic interval and mortality among patients receiving hemodialysis. N Engl J Med. 2011;365(12):1099–107. https://doi.org/10.1056/NEJMoa1103313.
30. Karnik JA, Young BS, Lew NL, et al. Cardiac arrest and sudden death in dialysis units. Kidney Int. 2001;60(1):350–7. https://doi.org/10.1046/j.1523-1755.2001.00806.x.
31. Jadoul M, Thumma J, Fuller DS, et al. Modifiable practices associated with sudden death among hemodialysis patients in the Dialysis Outcomes and Practice Patterns Study. Clin J Am Soc Nephrol. 2012;7(5):765–74. https://doi.org/10.2215/CJN.08850811.
32. Miller JE, Kovesdy CP, Norris KC, et al. Association of cumulatively low or high serum calcium levels with mortality in long-term hemodialysis patients. Am J Nephrol. 2010;32(5):403–13. https://doi.org/10.1159/000319861.
33. Pun PH, Horton JR, Middleton JP. Dialysate calcium concentration and the risk of sudden cardiac arrest in hemodialysis patients. Clin J Am Soc Nephrol. 2013;8(5):797–803. https://doi.org/10.2215/CJN.10000912.
34. Pun PH, Abdalla S, Block GA, et al. Cinacalcet, dialysate calcium concentration, and cardiovascular events in the EVOLVE trial. Hemodial Int. 2016;20(3):421–31. https://doi.org/10.1111/hdi.12382.
35. Rhee CM, Chou JA, Kalantar-Zadeh K. Dialysis prescription and sudden death. Semin Nephrol. 2018;38(6):570–81. https://doi.org/10.1016/j.semnephrol.2018.08.003.

36. Wu DY, Shinaberger CS, Regidor DL, McAllister CJ, Kopple JD, Kalantar-Zadeh K. Association between serum bicarbonate and death in hemodialysis patients: is it better to be acidotic or alkalotic? Clin J Am Soc Nephrol. 2006;1(1):70–8. https://doi.org/10.2215/CJN.00010505.
37. Bommer J, Locatelli F, Satayathum S, et al. Association of predialysis serum bicarbonate levels with risk of mortality and hospitalization in the Dialysis Outcomes and Practice Patterns Study (DOPPS). Am J Kidney Dis. 2004;44(4):661–71. (https://www.ncbi.nlm.nih.gov/pubmed/15384017).
38. Tentori F, Karaboyas A, Robinson BM, et al. Association of dialysate bicarbonate concentration with mortality in the Dialysis Outcomes and Practice Patterns Study (DOPPS). Am J Kidney Dis. 2013;62(4):738–46. https://doi.org/10.1053/j.ajkd.2013.03.035.
39. Correa S, Scovner KM, Tumlin JA, et al. Electrolyte changes in contemporary hemodialysis: a secondary analysis of the monitoring in dialysis (MiD) study. Kidney360. 2021;2(4):695–707. https://doi.org/10.34067/kid.0007452020.
40. Rogovoy NM, Howell SJ, Lee TL, et al. Hemodialysis procedure-associated autonomic imbalance and cardiac arrhythmias: insights from continuous 14-day ECG monitoring. J Am Heart Assoc. 2019;8(19):e013748. https://doi.org/10.1161/JAHA.119.013748.
41. Kaplan R, Passman R. Defibrillators don't deliver in dialysis. Circulation. 2019;139(23):2639–41. https://doi.org/10.1161/CIRCULATIONAHA.119.040504.
42. Buiten MS, de Bie MK, Rotmans JI, et al. The dialysis procedure as a trigger for atrial fibrillation: new insights in the development of atrial fibrillation in dialysis patients. Heart. 2014;100(9):685–90. https://doi.org/10.1136/heartjnl-2013-305,417.
43. Zoccali C, Mallamaci F, Parlongo S, et al. Plasma norepinephrine predicts survival and incident cardiovascular events in patients with end-stage renal disease. Circulation. 2002;105(11):1354–9. https://doi.org/10.1161/hc1102.105261.
44. Oikawa K, Ishihara R, Maeda T, et al. Prognostic value of heart rate variability in patients with renal failure on hemodialysis. Int J Cardiol. 2009;131(3):370–7. https://doi.org/10.1016/j.ijcard.2007.10.033.
45. Nishimura M, Tokoro T, Nishida M, et al. Sympathetic overactivity and sudden cardiac death among hemodialysis patients with left ventricular hypertrophy. Int J Cardiol. 2010;142(1):80–6. https://doi.org/10.1016/j.ijcard.2008.12.104.
46. Waks JW, Tereshchenko LG, Parekh RS. Electrocardiographic predictors of mortality and sudden cardiac death in patients with end stage renal disease on hemodialysis. J Electrocardiol. 2016;49(6):848–54. https://doi.org/10.1016/j.jelectrocard.2016.07.020.
47. Genovesi S, Rossi E, Nava M, et al. A case series of chronic haemodialysis patients: mortality, sudden death, and QT interval. Europace. 2013;15(7):1025–33. https://doi.org/10.1093/europace/eus412.
48. Hage FG, de Mattos AM, Khamash H, Mehta S, Warnock D, Iskandrian AE. QT prolongation is an independent predictor of mortality in end-stage renal disease. Clin Cardiol. 2010;33(6):361–6. https://doi.org/10.1002/clc.20768.
49. Oehler A, Feldman T, Henrikson CA, Tereshchenko LG. QRS-T angle: a review. Ann Noninvasive Electrocardiol. 2014;19(6):534–42. https://doi.org/10.1111/anec.12206.
50. de Bie MK, Koopman MG, Gaasbeek A, et al. Incremental prognostic value of an abnormal baseline spatial QRS-T angle in chronic dialysis patients. Europace. 2013;15(2):290–6. https://doi.org/10.1093/europace/eus306.
51. Tereshchenko LG, Kim ED, Oehler A, et al. Electrophysiologic substrate and risk of mortality in incident hemodialysis. J Am Soc Nephrol. 2016;27(11):3413–20. https://doi.org/10.1681/ASN.2015080916.
52. Shah NR, Charytan DM, Murthy VL, et al. Prognostic value of coronary flow reserve in patients with dialysis-dependent ESRD. J Am Soc Nephrol. 2016;27(6):1823–9. https://doi.org/10.1681/ASN.2015030301.

53. Murthy VL, Naya M, Foster CR, et al. Association between coronary vascular dysfunction and cardiac mortality in patients with and without diabetes mellitus. Circulation. 2012;126(15):1858–68. https://doi.org/10.1161/CIRCULATIONAHA.112.120402.
54. Pun PH, Al-Khatib SM. Implantable defibrillators for primary prevention of sudden death in patients on dialysis. Am J Kidney Dis. 2019;74(6):857–60. https://doi.org/10.1053/j.ajkd.2019.05.002.
55. Charytan DM, Patrick AR, Liu J, et al. Trends in the use and outcomes of implantable cardioverter-defibrillators in patients undergoing dialysis in the United States. Am J Kidney Dis. 2011;58(3):409–17. https://doi.org/10.1053/j.ajkd.2011.03.026.
56. Jukema JW, Timal RJ, Rotmans JI, et al. Prophylactic use of implantable cardioverter-defibrillators in the prevention of sudden cardiac death in dialysis patients. Circulation. 2019;139(23):2628–38. https://doi.org/10.1161/CIRCULATIONAHA.119.039818.
57. Burlacu A, Iftene A, Jugrin D, et al. Using artificial intelligence resources in dialysis and kidney transplant patients: a literature review. Biomed Res Int. 2020;2020:9867872. https://doi.org/10.1155/2020/9867872.
58. Akbilgic O, Obi Y, Potukuchi PK, et al. Machine learning to identify dialysis patients at high death risk. Kidney Int Rep. 2019;4(9):1219–29. https://doi.org/10.1016/j.ekir.2019.06.009.
59. https://arxiv.org/pdf/1707.01836.pdf.
60. Galloway CD, Valys AV, Shreibati JB, et al. Development and validation of a deep-learning model to screen for hyperkalemia from the electrocardiogram. JAMA Cardiol. 2019;4(5):428–36. https://doi.org/10.1001/jamacardio.2019.0640.
61. Yasin OZ, Attia Z, Dillon JJ, et al. Noninvasive blood potassium measurement using signal-processed, single-lead ECG acquired from a handheld smartphone. J Electrocardiol. 2017;50(5):620–5. https://doi.org/10.1016/j.jelectrocard.2017.06.008.

Chapter 16
Current and Future Technologies to Enhance Acceptance of Peritoneal Dialysis

Aditya Jain and Jaime Uribarri

Introduction

Compared to hemodialysis (HD), peritoneal dialysis (PD) offers improved quality of life, better preservation of residual renal function (RRF), and lower economic cost. The ballooning costs of healthcare, particularly in the USA, have driven the recent enthusiasm to increase the utilization of PD. To achieve this goal, innovation is critical in the long-term success of PD. In this chapter, we will review key advancements in PD.

The Current Use of Cyclers in PD

Patients who select PD for renal replacement therapy have two options: (1) continuous ambulatory PD (CAPD) where the patient performs manual exchanges throughout the day; or (2) automated PD (APD) or continuous cycling peritoneal dialysis (CCPD) where the patient uses a cycler machine.

APD is typically performed at night when the patient sleeps but can be done during the daytime. To perform APD, a patient will first connect to the cycler machine via their PD catheter. Their PD prescription is preprogrammed with the following components: (1) total treatment time; (2) total treatment volume; (3) number of exchanges or cycles; (4) fill volume per cycle; (5) last fill; and (6) tidal PD (Table 16.1). These variables are customized for each patient. Parameters for minimum and maximum dwell volume, drain volume, and drain time are also

A. Jain · J. Uribarri (✉)
Division of Nephrology, Icahn School of Medicine at Mount Sinai, New York, NY, USA
e-mail: Jaime.Uribarri@mountsinai.org

S. J. Saggi, M. O. Salifu (eds.), *Technological Advances in Care of Patients with Kidney Diseases*, https://doi.org/10.1007/978-3-031-11942-2_16

Table 16.1 Components of APD cycler prescription

Total treatment time
Total treatment volume
Number of exchanges
Fill volume per cycler
Strength of dextrose solution
Last fill
Tidal exchanges

programmed and the machine will alarm if outside those parameters. Each exchange is a three-step process. The peritoneal cavity is first filled with dialysate which will dwell for prespecified time based on total treatment time. The dialysis effluent is then drained into a drain bag or directly into the sewer system. This process is repeated for the programmed number of cycles. At the end of the cycler treatment, there is an option for last fill which consists of additional fluid that dwells in the patient during the daytime. The patient can drain this fluid either manually during the day or, more commonly, at the beginning of the next APD treatment. The tidal PD features allows for an incomplete drain of the peritoneal cavity during each exchange and it can be utilized temporarily in patients who experience pain at the end of drain. The percent of fluid left during each exchange is programmed into the cycler machine. Tidal PD should be used sparingly as it reduces the overall efficacy of the exchanges.

Patients with higher RRF require less dialysis clearance and total therapy time. A patient started on APD therapy may require anywhere from 6 to 10 h on the cycler. As RRF declines, an increase in total dialysis therapy time is needed and typically achieved by adding a last fill. Calculating Kt/V of urea is used as a surrogate measure of dialysis adequacy and a low value (by convention, less than 1.70 per week) will prompt increase in dialysis time and/or volume of each dwell.

The required dwell time varies between patients and depends on their ability to transport small solutes across their peritoneal membrane. This is determined by performing a Peritoneal Equilibration Test (PET). Slow transporters typically require longer dwell times compared to fast transporters who require shorter dwell times. Studies have shown that long-term exposure to dextrose-containing PD solutions may result in faster transport status over time.

Candidates for PD therapy are offered either CAPD or APD therapy, although the latter is by far the most popular option in the USA at present [1]. Neither mode has been consistently superior in mortality, hospitalization rates, fluid leaks nor volume management. Therefore, patient preference is the primary factor in deciding the mode of therapy. A clinician can guide the patient by considering lifestyle factors such as employment, social, and family obligations.

The major advantage of APD is the reduced therapy burden and more dialysis-free time resulting in less disruption to daily life (Table 16.2). Additionally, there is less caregiver burden and potential risk of peritonitis due to reduced numbers of connections and disconnections compared to CAPD therapy [2–4]. However, other studies have suggested no improvement in rates of peritonitis with APD use [5].

Table 16.2 Selection of APD compared to CAPD therapy

Benefits	Drawbacks
Improved flexibility with family, social, and employment obligations	More complex and requires a machine
Increased dialysis-free time	Disturbed sleep due to being tethered to a machine and alarms
Decreased care partners burden	Travel is more complicated
Reduced intraperitoneal pressures and potential hernia formation	
More suitable for fast transporters	

Furthermore, it is unclear if patients on APD have better technique survival (i.e., retaining a patient on PD) compared to CAPD with studies yielding mixed results [6–9].

There are also several disadvantages of APD therapy. The increased complexity compared to CAPD requires more lengthy training which can be logistically challenging for some patients. For this reason, some patients prefer CAPD due to the lack of machinery and its simplicity. Interruptions in sleep can occur on APD when a patient must be tethered to a machine for long periods or with alarms. Finally, travel is more complicated with APD due to the logistics of transporting the cycler machine and therefore some patients will temporarily switch to CAPD when traveling.

History and Innovation in PD Cycler Technology

The use of cyclers at home to perform APD was introduced in the 1960s. Subsequent innovations in APD cyclers eventually produced quieter, smaller, and more efficient machines. The main benefit was the ability to perform intermittent PD either in the day or night rather than the burden of continuous exchanges throughout the day. A major milestone in the development of cycler technology occurred with the development of the Homechoice® cycler by Baxter in the 1990s followed by the Liberty® cycler by Fresenius in the 2000s introducing the ability to store and access treatment data via a memory card. This card allowed clinical teams to review treatments, troubleshoot problems, and review patient adherence.

Modern cycler machines including the Homechoice Claria and Amia (produced by Baxter) and Liberty Select (produced by Fresenius Medical Care) [10] introduced significant advancements with the ability for remote patient monitoring (RPM). These machines transmit data bidirectionally using a modem and cellular network. The treatment data is uploaded to a cloud-based internet platform such as Sharesource by Baxter [11]. These new technologies allow for much faster review of treatment data including prescriptions, peritoneal membrane tests, and dialysis adequacy.

RPM allows expedited troubleshooting of clinical issues and adjust prescriptions in real-time which provides several important benefits. Firstly, the patient saves time and money on transportation by avoiding physical travel to the clinic. Improved inventory management reduces the potential issues with delivery of supplies which can lead to disruptions in treatment. RPM allows timely assessment of problems in treatment and early intervention to potentially avoid emergency room visits or hospitalizations which lead to adverse outcomes [12]. It also simplifies review of patient adherence which is critical to the success of home dialysis ultimately improving patient retention on PD. RPM technology became particularly important and complemented the rise in telehealth use in home dialysis particularly during the COVID-19 pandemic when physical travel is risky.

Patients are responsible for entering daily vital signs such as blood pressure, weights, and heart rate pre- and post-treatment. On the Sharesource platform, the clinic team can review treatment alarms such as inappropriate low ultrafiltration volume, line occlusion, slow fill, and slow drain. Parameters for alarms are individualized to the patient. Reducing the number of alarms is important for patient quality of life such as improved sleep. Furthermore, improved patient satisfaction can improve patient retention and reduce burnout.

Selected Examples of Troubleshooting Using Sharesource

1. The patient reports having difficulty sleeping due to excessive alarms at night. On Sharesource, the clinical team notes that the patient has "line occlusion" alarms. The patient is brought into the clinic and the nurse notes the presence of large fibrin clots after using forceful flushing of the PD catheter. The patient is started on intraperitoneal heparin 500 units per liter of dialysate. On follow-up, the patient reports no further alarms during treatment.
2. During a remote PD monthly telehealth visit, a patient presents with worsening leg edema and hypertension. Treatment data is reviewed on Sharesource and the team determines that that patient needs increased ultrafiltration. The patient is started on higher dextrose concentration dialysate to increase ultrafiltration. One week later, the patient reports improved leg edema with improved blood pressure and lower weight noted on Sharesource.
3. A patient reports increased lethargy, poor appetite, and worsening pruritis. The team reviews his treatment data on Sharesource and his monthly labs. His standardized weekly Kt/V of urea is noted to be 1.3 (below the goal of $\geq$1.7). Additionally, the team notes a significant decline in renal Kt/V of urea and decreased urine output compared to 6 months ago. A last fill is added to his cycler prescription. On a follow-up visit 1 month later, the patient reports improved energy, appetite, and pruritis.

Innovation in Biocompatible PD Dialysate Solutions

There are significant morphological changes to the peritoneal membrane over time for patients on PD. This transformation results in the loss of the mesenchymal layer, submesothelial fibrosis with increased thickness, and neoangiogenesis [13, 14]. The long-term exposure of the peritoneal membrane to low-pH, high lactate, and high-dextrose containing solutions have been implicated in generating glucose degradation products (GDP) and, subsequently, advanced glycation end-products (AGEs). These molecules are associated with the formation of reactive oxidation species and chronic inflammation which damages the peritoneal membrane over time [15–17].

During the manufacture and sterilization process, solutions are required to be kept at a pH close to 5.5 to prevent caramelization of glucose [18]. Lower pH close to 3 has been found to result in the lowest production of GDPs [19] but is not feasible for routine clinical use. In the USA, lactate is typically added as a source of alkali instead of bicarbonate to allow for the presence of calcium and magnesium in the same compartment without risk of precipitation.

There is continued interest in the development of alternative biocompatible PD solutions which form less GDPs and AGEs and potentially better preserve the peritoneal membrane. Fresenius and Baxter have produced variations on biocompatible dialysate, but they have not been widely adopted. These solutions are stored in a dual-bag system, one with the glucose and the other one with the buffer, which allows heat sterilization at very low pH thus minimizing GDP formation [20]. In vitro and in vivo studies have shown reduced inflammation, fibrosis, and neoangiogenesis with their use [21, 22]. Clinical trials, however, have not shown preservation of residual renal function or long-term membrane preservation [23]. At present, dextrose remains the osmotic agent of choice in PD therapy with the option to use icodextrin, a glucose polymer, as a last fill or for the long nocturnal dwell in CAPD patients.

Addition of essential amino acids in dialysate has also been studied to address malnutrition in PD. Loss of protein and amino acids occurs in PD and can result in significant negative nitrogen balance over time unless the patient replaces losses with oral intake. Addition of amino acids to the PD solution will lead to their increased absorption and potentially increased protein synthesis. However, clinical trials did not show improved nutritional status of patients.

Generation of Individualized PD Fluid at Home

Conventional PD solutions which are composed of dextrose, electrolytes, and water pose several challenges. The shipping and disposal of bulky boxes (on average 40 boxes monthly weighing approximately 900 pounds) has substantial economic and environmental costs. For patients, the storage of PD supplies takes up large amounts of space which can be a significant barrier for patients living in small dwellings. This problem has been, in part, addressed for patients on home hemodialysis where dialysate can be generated at home using tap water. Similarly, in 2019, Baxter announced the start of a clinical trial for an on-demand PD solution system, but no further announcements have yet followed. The appealing possibility of generating individualized PD fluid at home and increasing patient access to PD therapy could transform patient care.

Future Developments

One of the greatest challenges in all forms of dialysis is the requirement that the patient must be tethered to a machine. To overcome this problem, there is intensive research and development for a wearable artificial kidney. There are several potential technologies in development to address this issue. One such device is the automated wearable artificial kidney (AWAK) using sorbent technology [24] which was developed by AWAK technologies and is currently undergoing clinical trials. The primary touted benefit of the AWAK device is the ability to continue PD without the need for a large bulky machine. Instead, the device is small and light enough for the patient to wear. The device is connected to a patient's PD catheter and 1–1.5 L tidal dialysate exchanges are performed with around 500 cc drained per exchange. Dialysate is regenerated using sorbent technology [25]. The ultrafiltrate would be collected either in a drain bag or routed to the patient urinary bladder. A small pilot study was performed on patients currently on conventional PD therapy that reportedly demonstrated that the AWAK device could effectively provide small solute clearance. The final study results are still pending.

Prevention of peritonitis is another substantial challenge that is the focus of future research. Peritonitis currently is the leading cause of technique failure resulting in transfer to HD. Improving our ability to screen and detect peritonitis earlier is critical so that antibiotics could be initiated prior to significant inflammation and damage to the peritoneal membrane. Several devices are currently being investigated to address this issue.

References

1. Rabindranath KS, et al. Continuous ambulatory peritoneal dialysis versus automated peritoneal dialysis for end-stage renal disease. Cochrane Database Syst Rev. 2007;(2):CD006515.
2. Roumeliotis A, et al. APD or CAPD: one glove does not fit all. Int Urol Nephrol. 2021;53(6):1149–60.
3. Holley JL, Bernardini J, Piraino B. Continuous cycling peritoneal dialysis is associated with lower rates of catheter infections than continuous ambulatory peritoneal dialysis. Am J Kidney Dis. 1990;16(2):133–6.

4. Brown MC, et al. Peritoneal dialysis-associated peritonitis rates and outcomes in a national cohort are not improving in the post-millennium (2000-2007). Perit Dial Int. 2011;31(6):639–50.
5. Lan PG, et al. The association between peritoneal dialysis modality and peritonitis. Clin J Am Soc Nephrol. 2014;9(6):1091–7.
6. de Fijter CW, et al. Clinical efficacy and morbidity associated with continuous cyclic compared with continuous ambulatory peritoneal dialysis. Ann Intern Med. 1994;120(4):264–71.
7. Mujais S, Story K. Patient and technique survival on peritoneal dialysis in patients with failed renal allograft: a case-control study. Kidney Int Suppl. 2006;103:S133–7.
8. Mehrotra R, et al. The outcomes of continuous ambulatory and automated peritoneal dialysis are similar. Kidney Int. 2009;76(1):97–107.
9. Johnson DW, et al. Superior survival of high transporters treated with automated versus continuous ambulatory peritoneal dialysis. Nephrol Dial Transplant. 2010;25(6):1973–9.
10. Fresenius Medical Care. 2021, May 25. https://fmcna.com/products/home-dialysis-equipment/liberty-select-cycler/.
11. Baxter Sharesource. May 25. https://www.baxter.com/healthcare-professionals/renal-care/sharesource-remote-patient-management.
12. Sanabria M, et al. Remote patient monitoring program in automated peritoneal dialysis: impact on hospitalizations. Perit Dial Int. 2019;39(5):472–8.
13. Williams JD, et al. Morphologic changes in the peritoneal membrane of patients with renal disease. J Am Soc Nephrol. 2002;13(2):470–9.
14. Mateijsen MA, et al. Vascular and interstitial changes in the peritoneum of CAPD patients with peritoneal sclerosis. Perit Dial Int. 1999;19(6):517–25.
15. Mahiout A, Ehlerding G, Brunkhorst R. Advanced glycation end-products in the peritoneal fluid and in the peritoneal membrane of continuous ambulant peritoneal dialysis patients. Nephrol Dial Transplant. 1996;11(Suppl 5):2–6.
16. De Vriese AS, et al. Inhibition of the interaction of AGE-RAGE prevents hyperglycemia-induced fibrosis of the peritoneal membrane. J Am Soc Nephrol. 2003;14(8):2109–18.
17. Tuncer M, et al. Chemical peritonitis associated with high dialysate acetaldehyde concentrations. Nephrol Dial Transplant. 2000;15(12):2037–40.
18. Rippe B, et al. Clinical and physiological effects of a new, less toxic and less acidic fluid for peritoneal dialysis. Perit Dial Int. 1997;17(1):27–34.
19. Erixon M, et al. Take care in how you store your PD fluids: actual temperature determines the balance between reactive and non-reactive GDPs. Perit Dial Int. 2005;25(6):583–90.
20. Passlick-Deetjen J, Lage C. Lactate-buffered and bicarbonate-buffered solutions with less glucose degradation products in a two-chamber system. Perit Dial Int. 2000;20(Suppl 2):S42–7.
21. Williams JD, et al. The euro-balance trial: the effect of a new biocompatible peritoneal dialysis fluid (balance) on the peritoneal membrane. Kidney Int. 2004;66(1):408–18.
22. Bartosova M, Schmitt CP. Biocompatible peritoneal dialysis: the target is still way off. Front Physiol. 2018;9:1853.
23. Fan SL, et al. Randomized controlled study of biocompatible peritoneal dialysis solutions: effect on residual renal function. Kidney Int. 2008;73(2):200–6.
24. AWAK Technologies. 2021, May 25. https://www.awak.com/technology.
25. Ronco C, Davenport A, Gura V. The future of the artificial kidney: moving towards wearable and miniaturized devices. Nefrologia. 2011;31(1):9–16.

Chapter 17
Project ECHO: Building Workforce Capacity to Improve Care for Patients with Kidney Disease

Emily Byers and Sanjeev Arora

Introduction

Across the USA, too many of the one in seven Americans who have chronic kidney disease [1] are not getting urgently needed care early enough to prevent end-stage renal disease [2–4]. Models based on health and nutrition survey data predict approximately half of U.S. adults age 30–64 will develop chronic kidney disease (CKD) in their lifetime [3]. Patients with early stage CKD require specialized testing and renal care to improve clinical outcomes and slow progression from early stage CKD to end-stage renal disease (ESRD), where renal replacement therapy (i.e., dialysis) is needed to perform renal functions in place of damaged kidneys [5]. Receiving specialized nephrology care earlier also increases patients' likelihood of receiving a kidney transplant [2]. Clinical guidelines recommend all patients with CKD receive care from a nephrologist and consult with a registered dietician by stages 4–5 of CKD. Unfortunately, 25–50% of pre-ESRD patients in the United States have never been evaluated by, or received care from, a nephrologist or other trained renal care provider [6].

Lack of access to specialty care disproportionately affects minority patients in rural areas, where demand for nephrologists is high, but supply three times less than in urban areas [7]. Rural residents are less likely to receive health screenings or

E. Byers (✉)
University of New Mexico Health Sciences Center ECHO Institute, University of New Mexico, Albuquerque, NM, USA
e-mail: elbyers@salud.unm.edu

S. Arora
University of New Mexico Health Sciences Center ECHO Institute, University of New Mexico, Albuquerque, NM, USA

University of New Mexico Health Sciences Center, Albuquerque, NM, USA
e-mail: sarora@salud.unm.edu

S. J. Saggi, M. O. Salifu (eds.), *Technological Advances in Care of Patients with Kidney Diseases*, https://doi.org/10.1007/978-3-031-11942-2_17

preventive education on CKD, and are less likely to have a dietician practicing in their communities [6]. CKD also disproportionately affects women [3], particularly rural women of color [1]. Eliminating racial and ethnic disparities across all stages of CKD was a stated goal of the U.S. government's public health strategic plan *Healthy People 2020* [8]. Regrettably, racial disparities and urban/rural disparities endure with life-threatening consequences [4]. Black patients are still 34% less likely to receive more than 12 months of pre-ESRD specialty care and 60% less likely to receive in-home hemodialysis compared to White patients [4, 7].

Lack of access to specialized medical care has burdened rural residents for decades, forcing patients to travel long distances to urban medical centers to receive complex treatments from doctors they do not know. Recently, however, urban communities have also experienced demand outstrip availability of renal replacement services (i.e., dialysis). The coronavirus disease 2019 (COVID-19) pandemic exposed health system vulnerabilities in rural and urban medical centers alike, including skilled workforce shortages, equipment shortages, infrastructure inadequacies, and planning failures that impeded delivery of lifesaving dialysis treatment [9–11]. Nearly nationwide surges in COVID-19 related hospital admissions quickly overtook ICU bed capacity [12]. Many rural hospitals then lost their safety net of being able to transfer patients with complex care needs to urban medical centers. In the USA, the estimated percentage of hospitalized COVID-19 patients suffering from acute kidney injury—a known risk factor for mortality from COVID-19—ranges from 15% to 50% by region [13, 14]. A study of Rhode Island Hospital's dialysis allocation plan found a number of issues impeding efficient delivery of renal replacement services, ranging from insufficient numbers of dialysis nurses and patient care technicians to lack of sinks in many ICU rooms preventing nurses from using reverse osmosis systems in-room to offer dialysis to quarantined patients [9]. Shortages of trained dialysis nurses are particularly burdensome to hospitals because they are required to be present during dialysis sessions to monitor patients and maintain equipment [9].

Prior to the pandemic, workforce shortages of patient care technicians, nurses, and nephrologists specializing in CKD and ESRD care vis-à-vis an aging U.S. population had already been identified as pending health system vulnerabilities [7, 15, 16]. Renal replacement service centers and providers must balance competing needs for equipment and trained staff to provide dialysis services to patients with acute kidney injury versus patients requiring maintenance dialysis services as part of their ongoing ESRD care plan. Frameworks for fairly allocating resources between acute and ESRD patients are currently under development [15]. The existing nephrology workforce, hospital internists, and generalist healthcare providers who treat ESRD require training on evolving clinical guidelines and ethical frameworks for allocating dialysis resources during public health emergencies.

Nephrology workforce shortages have been a source of concern for some time given the U.S' demographic evolution toward an aging population with complex care needs. Multiple health system stakeholders have called for greater cooperation between nephrology and critical care medicine, hospital-based and community nephrologists, and community dialysis units, as well as regional collaborations between clinicians at regional hospitals and outpatient facilities [5, 10, 13]. While the COVID-19 pandemic has created a surge of need for dialysis services and trained providers, it has also created obstacles to traditional methods for large-scale training of healthcare providers. Travel restrictions and bans on in-person gatherings have postponed many traditional continuing education opportunities, while some events and courses have transitioned to a virtual format with mixed results [17, 18]. Fortunately, a quality remote learning model exists for using virtual platforms to build and sustain professional knowledge networks for mentoring all sectors of the clinical and administrative healthcare workforce through sharing best practices for providing ESRD care to patients now and in the future.

This chapter discusses how Project ECHO (Extension for Community Health Outcomes)—a proven telementoring model for building workforce capacity and scaling best practices—can be adapted to improve outcomes for ESRD. A description of the ECHO model is accompanied a high-level overview of the steps to becoming an ECHO partner. Strategies for including patients as direct participants in nephrology ECHO programs conclude the chapter.

Project ECHO: Moving Knowledge, Not People

Project ECHO is an innovative iterative guided practice model for building workforce capacity among primary care providers (PCPs) through telementoring programs that move knowledge from urban academic medical centers or tertiary care centers to primary care clinics in remote and underserved areas. TeleECHO programs use case-based learning strategies similar to the medical school model for generalizing knowledge and developing expertise over time using real patient cases. Project ECHO uses a "hub and spoke" model where interdisciplinary teams of specialists at academic medical/tertiary care centers ("hubs") mentor cohorts of healthcare providers remotely using videoconferencing technology. Participants enroll in ECHO programs to develop professional competence to provide specialized medical screenings and treatments to patients at their local clinic ("spoke") while receiving ongoing case management support from the hub team. ECHO programs promote health equity by moving knowledge into rural and underserved communities where residents lack resources to make multiple trips to urban medical centers for evaluation and treatment.

Project ECHO was launched at the University of New Mexico in 2003 for training PCPs across New Mexico to provide hepatitis C (HCV) treatment to patients locally. By training rural PCPs to administer treatment, liver disease specialists reduce wait times for their appointments by 90%. ECHO has allowed specialists to prioritize appointments for complex cases while co-managing routine cases alongside ECHO program participants as they continue building expertise and confidence to provide specialized treatments alone.

Since that first program began, Project ECHO has been adapted to train health workers on over 70 medical conditions and public health topics. Over 520 partner organizations have become ECHO partner hubs, offering more than 960 programs across 45 countries.[1] Project ECHO's effectiveness is tested and confirmed through a robust body of peer-reviewed research, including more than 335 academic publications demonstrating provider and patient outcomes. A 2011 study published in the *New England Journal of Medicine* found that ECHO-trained doctors in rural New Mexico achieved HCV cure rates (SVR-12) equal to, or slightly better than, liver disease specialists at the UNM specialty clinic [19]. ECHO's origin story parallels current workforce issues facing nephrology in that there are more people suffering from kidney disease than the existing number of specialists can manage, and health disparities exist between the treatment options and outcomes for white patients and minority patients. Rural residents are often unaware they have chronic kidney disease, which denies them the opportunity to educate themselves or talk with their doctor about best practices for receiving early treatments that could prevent irreversible and life-threatening damage from occurring. Though Project ECHO is relatively new to the nephrology subdiscipline, comparable evidence of improved outcomes exists for patients with complex, chronic conditions including diabetes, cancer, and HIV infection [20–23].

ESRD is an ideal topic for implementing Project ECHO because the symptoms and treatment are complex to manage and patients with ESRD often have comorbid conditions (e.g., diabetes) that require input from multiple specialists to maximize outcomes. Patients with ESRD also commonly suffer from mental health issues like depression that can adversely affect their treatment adherence or dissuade them from pursuing a transplant. A nephrology ECHO program gives PCPs the opportunity to raise mental health issues or ask about symptoms related to comorbid conditions. The hub team facilitates group discussion based on ECHO's "all teach, all learn" commitment to group problem solving prior to treatment recommendations (Fig. 17.1). Presenting real patient cases empowers ECHO participants to gain confidence and assume responsibility for managing complex patients. When not presenting cares, ECHO providers continue acquiring generalizable knowledge through participation during group discussion.

ECHO programs serve as catalysts for overcoming translational gaps from research to practice [24]. To date, the USA has not experienced widescale adoption of pre-emptive kidney transplants, nor in-home hemodialysis as the preferred treatment option for patients with ESRD. In 2019, the U.S. Department of Health and Human Services and the U.S. Centers for Medicare & Medicaid Services created new payment models designed to facilitate in-home hemodialysis as the preferred treatment mechanism. Studies suggest low rates of adoption are attributable both to a lack of patient education on available treatment options, and to inadequate access to kidney disease testing and treatment prior before patients' health conditions reach ESRD [25]. Approximately 35% of current patients experience dialysis for the first time in a medical office or hospital, having had no prior diagnosis of chronic kidney disease many start dialysis in the hospital following grave health emergencies [26].

[1] https://hsc.unm.edu/echo/data-marketplace/interactive-dashboards/.

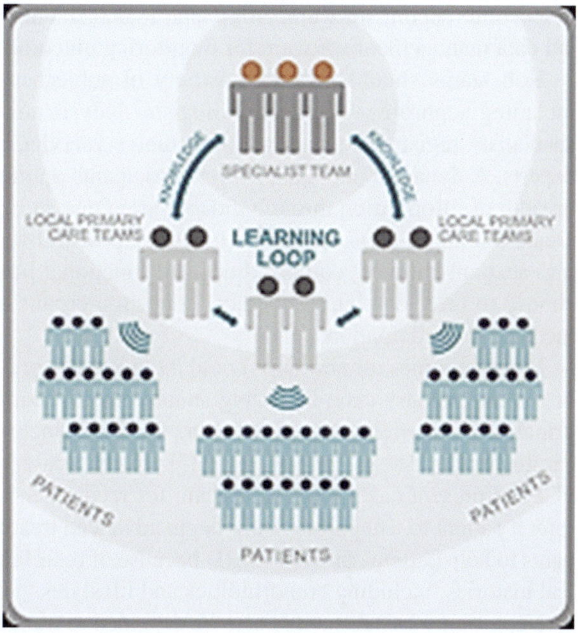

Fig. 17.1 The ECHO model moves life-saving knowledge out into local communities to increase the number of patients receiving care

To overcome provider hesitancy and lack of patient education regarding home hemodialysis treatments, Chan et al. advocated implementing a pilot Project ECHO where high performing home dialysis serve as hubs to mentor smaller home dialysis units on best practices [25]. At present, there are many opportunities for prospective hubs to democratize knowledge and improve outcomes for patients with ESRD by training local care teams to implement evidence-based practices for treating ESRD.

Becoming a Project ECHO Nephrology Hub

Organizations interested in becoming an ECHO hub are invited to attend an ECHO Immersion training at no cost to learn in-depth about the ECHO model and the steps for becoming an official ECHO replicating partner. Virtual immersion trainings are currently available once a month to accommodate travel restrictions.[2] ECHO immersion provides in-depth training on the ECHO model and offers organizations the opportunity to work with ECHO Institute staff on designing and launching an ECHO program. Immersion training covers program operations, securing funding, spoke recruitment and retention, developing curricula, and monitoring and evaluation strategies. Following Immersion training, organizations sign partnership documents with the ECHO Institute and receive technical support and access to

[2] https://hsc.unm.edu/echo/get-involved/start-a-hub/immersion-training.html.

videoconferencing software, Box cloud management software, and ECHO's internal data management software for monitoring outcomes.

Hub teams should include a variety of subject-matter experts and clinicians including nephrologists, endocrinologists, dialysis nurses, psychiatrists, transplant specialists, registered dieticians, home dialysis service providers, and palliative care experts. A dynamic hub team offers participants a unique opportunity to receive a breadth of information through didactic trainings and group discussion, and to co-create treatment plans under the mentorship of a diverse panel of experts, taking into account patients' comorbidities and functional limitations. Some ECHO hubs choose to offer continuing medical education credits at no cost to participants to incentivize participation.

Program topics for new hubs could include CKD prevention and detection as part of routine primary care, including annual serum creatinine screenings and routine urinalysis for patients with risk factors for CKD, including diabetes, hypertension, cardiovascular disease, and obesity [27]. ECHO's case-based learning format allows PCPs to present cases to the hub team for recommendations on the appropriate to refer a patient to a nephrologist to begin advanced treatment. PCPs are ideal participants to help patients prevent ESRD because of their familiarity with patients' medical histories, including comorbidities and lifestyles.

Nephrology ECHOs could also be designed to train nephrologists at community dialysis centers to identify patients who are likely good candidates for kidney transplantation. Under the current system, patients must travel to academic medical centers for evaluation by a transplant team including a transplant surgeon, a transplant nephrologist (healthcare provider specializing in the treatment of the kidneys), one or more transplant nurses, a social worker, and a psychiatrist or psychologist. The ECHO model eliminates travel burdens and wait times by allowing a nephrologist at a community dialysis center to present the patient's case to the specialist hub team who can help participants develop expertise in evaluating suitable transplant candidates and recommend next steps for eligible patients. ECHO hubs training providers at community dialysis centers should also consider adding quality improvement ECHO programs to train multiple centers to implement best practices.

When managed correctly, in-home hemodialysis has been shown to extend patients' lives and improve chances of remaining employed and other quality of life measures [28]. ECHO programs can improve the quality of in-home hemodialysis care by providing the virtual platform to expand awareness of the treatment option and the expertise to increase adoption of the procedure as the standard treatment option for patients with ESRD. ECHO hub teams can work closely with state and federal health agencies to promote the best practice and educate spoke staff on policy changes related to insurance and cost reimbursement for this service now and in the years to come. ECHO hub teams can also work with providers to train caregivers to assist patients with the procedure. To end health disparities, ECHO programs can work with community stakeholders, social service providers, and a variety of healthcare employees to overcome patient barriers to accessing in-home hemodialysis, lack of knowledge or exposure to the procedure and perceived complexity of this modality [25, 28].

The following examples highlight various ways that ECHO programs have been customized to meet needs of their communities:

- *VA kidney SCAN-ECHO*: The Department of Veterans' Affairs' (VA) Specialty Care Access Network-Extension for Community Health Care Outcomes (SCAN-ECHO) enables primary care clinics serving veterans to receive specialized nephrology training. Specialists at regional VA medical clinics form the hub team and remotely mentor PCPs at their local clinics. Session topics include diabetic and hypertension guidelines, primary care for patients with ESRD, and serious side effects including anemia and hyperkalemia [29]. In the early stages of Kidney SCAN-ECHO, program teams made socialization visits to prospective spoke cites to build enthusiasm for the program. Like many ECHO programs, SCAN-ECHO offered continuing medical education credits to providers at no cost to incentivize participation [29].
- *SHOW-ME KIDNEY DISEASE ECHO*: The University of Missouri's SHOW-ME Kidney Disease ECHO improves PCPs' ability to screen and identify patients at risk for kidney disease and mentors them on strategies to educate patients. This ECHO program also mentors PCPs on best practices for managing chronic kidney disease and ESRD patients with complex, chronic conditions, while emphasizing the role of the physician in empowering patients to practice self-management of their medication regimens. Beyond co-managing patients with stable conditions, SHOW-ME ECHO trains providers on recognizing signs that a patient should be referred to a nephrologist to prepare for or treat existing ESRD, or begin their search for a kidney transplant.
- *Endo ECHO*: Endo ECHO was launched at the University of New Mexico in partnership with ten federally qualified healthcare centers (FHQCs) statewide to implement best practices for improving outcomes among patients with complex diabetes. Participant teams were dyads consisting of one PCP and a community health worker (CHW). The multidisciplinary hub team included experts in endocrinology, nephology, psychiatry, social work, and certified diabetes educators. Participants attended weekly virtual teleECHO sessions consisting of didactic presentations and case presentations.

Patients of ECHO-trained PCPs had much in common with patients who have chronic kidney disease or ESRD. Over half were female, and over 60% self-identified as a racial or ethnic minority. The majority of patients reported at least one co-morbidity to their complex diabetes diagnosis, with nearly 70% having high blood pressure and over 40% suffering from depression. The clearest parallel between these endocrinology patients and typical kidney disease patients is that at baseline, fewer than 35% of enrolled patients had ever seen an endocrinologist.

A team of evaluators at New York University worked with CHWs to evaluate patient health outcomes using survey questions adapted from a variety of standardized assessments measuring health and well-being outcomes among patients with diabetes [22]. Patients were interviewed in person at the start of the program and again by telephone at the 1-year mark [30]. The number of patients who reported delays in accessing medical care decreased over the first year and the number of patients reporting four or more visits to their PCP increased from 55% to 72% [30]. Patients reported that they received significantly more foot exams, eye exams, screenings for smoking status, and more frequent HbA1c checks during their year of program participation [30]. Moreover, Endo ECHO participating physicians significantly increased self-efficacy to treat complex diabetes and comorbid conditions by 60%, while CHW's reported a 130% increase in self-efficacy to monitor and support patients' progress [31].

Prospective partners may find the Endo ECHO model contains a blueprint for improving outcomes for patients with ESRD, in no small part because of the high percentage of co-morbidity between ESRD and complex diabetes. With best practices recommending home hemodialysis as the preferred treatment method for ESRD, nephrology hubs could add additional teleECHO sessions training PCPs to educate their patients on managing various aspects of diabetes testing and treatment from home.

Discussion

Project ECHO is a promising healthcare intervention for building workforce capacity and promoting best practices for treating patients with ESRD. Nephrology is a very compatible with the components of the ECHO model in that it is complex and life threatening, with evolving treatments requiring healthcare providers to continue their professional learning to adopt best practices. By attending a virtual or in-person ECHO Immersion training, prospective partners receive in-depth training on the ECHO model at no cost, as well as support from the ECHO Institute training team on the necessary components for launching an ECHO hub. ESRD cases are expected to grow quickly as the U.S. population ages—a demand that lengthy medical education programs cannot meet expeditiously. Moreover, traditional methods of training more nephrologists may not solve the problem, as experts tend to reside close to renal disease specialty clinics in urban centers far away from the rural patients who need their services. By moving knowledge, not people, ECHO can help by training generalist healthcare providers on best practices, including preemptive transplants and home-based dialysis, to end health disparities and improve quality of life for patients with ESRD everywhere.

References

1. Chronic kidney disease basics | Chronic kidney disease initiative | CDC. Published March 9, 2021. https://www.cdc.gov/kidneydisease/basics.html. Accessed 14 Mar 2021.
2. Gillespie BW, Morgenstern H, Hedgeman E, et al. Nephrology care prior to end-stage renal disease and outcomes among new ESRD patients in the USA. Clin Kidney J. 2015;8(6):772–80. https://doi.org/10.1093/ckj/sfv103.

3. Hoerger TJ, Simpson SA, Yarnoff BO, et al. The future burden of CKD in the United States: a simulation model for the CDC CKD initiative. Am J Kidney Dis. 2015;65(3):403–11. https://doi.org/10.1053/j.ajkd.2014.09.023.
4. Norris KC, Williams SF, Rhee CM, et al. Hemodialysis disparities in African Americans: the deeply integrated concept of race in the social fabric of our society. Semin Dial. 2017;30(3):213–23. https://doi.org/10.1111/sdi.12589.
5. Wouters OJ, O'Donoghue DJ, Ritchie J, Kanavos PG, Narva AS. Early chronic kidney disease: diagnosis, management and models of care. Nat Rev Nephrol. 2015;11(8):491–502. https://doi.org/10.1038/nrneph.2015.85.
6. Yan G, Cheung AK, Ma JZ, et al. The associations between race and geographic area and quality-of-care indicators in patients approaching ESRD. Clin J Am Soc Nephrol. 2013;8(4):610–8. https://doi.org/10.2215/CJN.07780812.
7. Mehrotra R, Shaffer RN, Molitoris BA. Implications of a nephrology workforce shortage for dialysis patient care. Semin Dial. 2011;24(3):275–7. https://doi.org/10.1111/j.1525-139X.2011.00933.x.
8. U.S. Department of Health and Human Services. Access to Health Services | Healthy People 2020. Office of Disease Prevention and Health Promotion; 2021. https://www.healthypeople.gov/2020/leading-health-indicators/2020-lhi-topics/Access-to-Health-Services/data. Accessed 14 Mar 2021.
9. Mitchell KR, Bomm A, Shea BS, Shemin D, Bayliss G. Inpatient dialysis planning during the COVID-19 pandemic: a single-center experience and review of the literature. Int J Nephrol Renovasc Dis. 2020;13:253–9. https://doi.org/10.2147/IJNRD.S275075.
10. Peterson-Kaiser Family Foundation P. Interactive maps highlight urban-rural differences in hospital bed capacity. KFF Newsroom. Published April 23, 2020. https://www.kff.org/health-costs/press-release/interactive-maps-highlight-urban-rural-differences-in-hospital-bed-capacity/. Accessed 10 June 2020.
11. Fast facts on U.S. Hospitals. 2020. AHA. https://www.aha.org/statistics/fast-facts-us-hospitals. Accessed 10 June 2020.
12. CDC. Rural communities: COVID-19 and your health. Centers for Disease Control and Prevention. Published January 21, 2021. Accessed 14 Mar 2021. https://www.cdc.gov/coronavirus/2019-ncov/need-extra-precautions/other-at-risk-populations/rural-communities.html#:~:text=Many%20rural%20hospitals%20have%20a,broadband%20and%20internet%20communications.
13. Adapa S, Aeddula NR, Konala VM, et al. COVID-19 and renal failure: challenges in the delivery of renal replacement therapy. J Clin Med Res. 2020;12(5):276–85. https://doi.org/10.14740/jocmr4160.
14. Meeting the demand for renal replacement therapy during the COVID-19 pandemic: a manufacturer's perspective | American Society of Nephrology. https://kidney360.asnjournals.org/content/2/2/350. Accessed 14 Mar 2021.
15. Carson RC, Forzley B, Thomas S, et al. Balancing the needs of acute and maintenance dialysis patients during the COVID-19 pandemic: a proposed ethical framework for dialysis allocation. Clin J Am Soc Nephrol. 2021;16(7):1122–30. https://doi.org/10.2215/CJN.07460520.
16. Salsberg E, Quigley L, Mehfoud N, Masselink L, Collins A. The U.S. adult nephrology workforce 2016: developments and trends. American Society of Nephrology; 2016. https://www.asn-online.org/education/training/workforce/Nephrology_Workforce_Study_Report_2016.pdf. Accessed 19 Mar 2021.
17. Jeyakumar Y, Sharma D, Sirianni G, Nyhof-Young J, Otremba M, Leung F-H. Limitations in virtual clinical skills education for medical students during COVID-19. Can Med Educ J. 2020;11(6):e165–6. https://doi.org/10.36834/cmej.70240.
18. Sethi RK, Nemani V, Shaffrey C, Lenke L, Sponseller P. Reimagining medical conferences for a virtual setting. Harvard Business Review; 2020. Published online December 10, 2020. https://hbr.org/2020/12/reimagining-medical-conferences-for-a-virtual-setting. Accessed 14 Mar 2021

19. Arora S, Thornton K, Murata G, et al. Outcomes of treatment for hepatitis C virus infection by primary care providers. N Engl J Med. 2011;364(23):2199–207. https://doi.org/10.1056/NEJMoa1009370.
20. Ness TE, Annese MF, Martinez-Paz N, Unruh KT, Scott JD, Wood BR. Using an innovative telehealth model to support community providers who deliver perinatal HIV care. AIDS Educ Prev. 2017;29(6):516–26. https://doi.org/10.1521/aeap.2017.29.6.516.
21. Bikinesi L, O'Brien G, Roscoe C, et al. Implementation and evaluation of a project ECHO telementoring program for the Namibian HIV workforce. Hum Resour Health. 2020;18(1):1–10.
22. Paul M, Davila Saad A, Billings J, Blecker S, Bouchonville MF, Berry C. MON-190 Endo ECHO improves patient-reported measures of access to care, health care quality, self-care behaviors, and overall quality of life for patients with complex diabetes in medically underserved areas of New Mexico. J Endocr Soc. 2019;3(Suppl 1). https://doi.org/10.1210/js.2019-MON-190.
23. Oliver K, Beskin K, Noonan L, Shah A, Perkins R, Humiston S. A quality improvement learning collaborative for human papillomavirus vaccination. Pediatr Qual Saf. 2020;6(1):e377. https://doi.org/10.1097/pq9.0000000000000377.
24. Morris ZS, Wooding S, Grant J. The answer is 17 years, what is the question: understanding time lags in translational research. J R Soc Med. 2011;104(12):510–20. https://doi.org/10.1258/jrsm.2011.110180.
25. Chan CT, Collins K, Ditschman EP, et al. Overcoming barriers for uptake and continued use of home dialysis: an NKF-KDOQI conference report. Am J Kidney Dis. 2020;75(6):926–34. https://doi.org/10.1053/j.ajkd.2019.11.007.
26. Saran R, Robinson B, Abbott KC, et al. US renal data system 2018 annual data report: epidemiology of kidney disease in the United States. Am J Kidney Dis. 2019;73(3, Supplement 1):A7–8. https://doi.org/10.1053/j.ajkd.2019.01.001.
27. Gaitonde DY, Cook DL, Rivera IM. Chronic kidney disease: detection and evaluation. Am Fam Physician. 2017;96(12):776–83. https://www.aafp.org/afp/2017/1215/p776.html. Accessed 29 Mar 2021.
28. Walker RC, Howard K, Morton RL. Home hemodialysis: a comprehensive review of patient-centered and economic considerations. Clinicoecon Outcomes Res. 2017;9:149–61. https://doi.org/10.2147/CEOR.S69340.
29. Koraishy FM, Rohatgi R. Telenephrology: an emerging platform for delivering renal health care. Am J Kidney Dis. 2020;76(3):417–26. https://doi.org/10.1053/j.ajkd.2020.02.442.
30. Paul MM, Saad AD, Billings J, et al. A telementoring intervention leads to improvements in self-reported measures of health care access and quality among patients with complex diabetes. J Health Care Poor Underserved. 2020;31(3):1124–33. https://doi.org/10.1353/hpu.2020.0085.
31. Bouchonville MF, Hager BW, Kirk JB, Qualls CR, Arora S. Endo ECHO improves primary care provider and community health worker self-efficacy in complex diabetes management in medically underserved communities. Endocr Pract. 2018;24(1):40–6. https://doi.org/10.4158/EP-2017-0079.

Chapter 18
Use of Artificial Intelligence/Machine Learning for Individualization of Drug Dosing in Dialysis Patients

Adam E. Gaweda, George R. Aronoff, and Michael E. Brier

Artificial intelligence (AI) is the term applied to computers and programs which attempt to mimic the decision-making capabilities of humans. Machine learning is a subset of artificial intelligence and is the study of computer algorithms that improve performance of a specific task following exposure to data. Both of these techniques have recently been "discovered" in the nephrology literature as evidenced by several publications in leading nephrology journals [1–5]. These applications of artificial intelligence have been applied to the prediction of acute kidney injury, mortality, nephropathology, and immune fingerprinting. The 2019 review by Lemley focuses on the application of exotic technologies that have been adopted by the nephrology community. In his review he introduces us to the concept of "deep learning" a type of artificial neural network used to analyze large data sets. These types of approaches have been historically utilized in image processing but were recently applied to the prediction of acute kidney injury [6]. These recent applications of artificial intelligence in nephrology have treated the subject as one of recent origin. However, one of the first reviews of artificial intelligence in nephrology was published in 1987 [7] following the proliferation of this topic in the engineering literature in the 1970s. The utility of an AI approach in prediction can be questioned

A. E. Gaweda
Department of Medicine, University of Louisville, Louisville, KY, USA
e-mail: adam.gaweda@louisville.edu

G. R. Aronoff
DaVita Kidney Care, Denver, CO, USA
e-mail: George.aronoff@louisville.edu

M. E. Brier (✉)
Department of Medicine, University of Louisville, Louisville, KY, USA

Robley Rex Veterans Administration Medical Center, Louisville, KY, USA
e-mail: michael.brier@louisville.edu

S. J. Saggi, M. O. Salifu (eds.), *Technological Advances in Care of Patients with Kidney Diseases*, https://doi.org/10.1007/978-3-031-11942-2_18

in some of the recent publications where no clear advantage to that approach was demonstrated [6]. One area that has shown utility is using artificial intelligence in the individualization of drug dosing.

Despite numerous publications on the impact of chronic kidney disease on the clearance of a drug in patients and the compilation of that information into a compendium [8], drug dosing is still a trial and error approach. Historically, the knowledge of how to dose a drug was privy to the individual that developed that knowledge. In 1844 a dentist by the name of Horace Wells experimented with the delivery of nitrous oxide to patients for dental extraction. Dr. Wells developed the idea of using nitrous oxide as an anesthetic agent following the attendance of a laughing gas show. Wells perfected the administration of nitrous oxide over the tooth extraction in 15 patients. He proceeded to demonstrate the procedure before a large audience at Massachusetts Gen. hospital in February 1845. Unfortunately, the gasbag was mistakenly withdrawn much too soon as admitted by Wells and the patient reported some pain associated with the procedure. Since there were no other volunteers the demonstration concluded, and several attendees commented that it was a humbug affair. After this demonstration Wells began testing chloroform as a dental anesthetic before taking his own life. Thus, ended any accumulated knowledge on the use of both nitrous oxide and chloroform as a dental anesthetic.

The same process that Horace Wells performed when evaluating nitrous oxide as a dental anesthetic is performed daily by physicians where they observe and follow that up with a recommendation. In the case of a differential diagnosis, the patient may present with dysuria and pyuria and the physician might conclude that the patient has cystitis. However, if the patient presents with dysuria and pyuria associated with fever and flank pain then the physician might conclude that the patient has pyelonephritis. When dosing a drug, the physician will make a recommendation for a specific drug and administration schedule and at an appropriate later time will observe the patient for a response. Depending on the nature of the response the physician may increase or decrease the drug dose or switch to a new drug.

The knowledge that goes into the selection of that first dose is contained in the field of pharmacokinetics and pharmacodynamics. Pharmacokinetics is the study of the absorption, distribution, metabolism, and elimination of the drug. Pharmacodynamics is the study of the time course of the effect of the drug. During the process of bringing a new drug to market the pharmaceutical manufacturer must provide this information in the package insert for the selection of the proper dose amount. The package insert may also contain information on how to adjust the dose. But often, dose adjustment is left to the physician. These approaches are often based on the mean response in a population of patients and can be successful for many drugs that have the following qualities: (1) follow an uncomplicated disposition, (2) demonstrate the variability in the pharmacokinetics and pharmacodynamics, (3) exhibit a wide therapeutic window, and (4) have a strong relationship between blood levels and drug effect. The problem arises in those patients that are not near the population mean response. Physicians treat individual patients and not populations.

The question then becomes can we do a better job of drug dosing beyond the information contained in the package insert. To answer this question, we can turn to the dialysis population where we have a drug that is routinely administered, doses are tracked, there is a definitive endpoint which is routinely monitored, and we have a narrow therapeutic range. The drug in question is that of erythropoietin (EPO). Problems associated with anemia management by the administration of exogenous EPO are multifactorial. The first problem is that the information in the package insert, although updated considering certain clinical trials and related adverse events, reflects the environment in which the agent was dosed over 30 years ago. The guidance for dosing EPO in the anemia of chronic kidney disease was vague enough that dialysis clinics needed to develop their own algorithm for individualizing EPO dosing. The resulting variability introduced by multiple dosing algorithms can be seen in Fig. 18.1. Despite all methods sharing a common goal of achieving a concentration of hemoglobin between 10 and 12 g/dL, each algorithm has a different mean hemoglobin achieved and vastly different variability surrounding that mean hemoglobin. This is an expected result since each algorithm was developed by a different individual or team of individuals that do not have a shared experience.

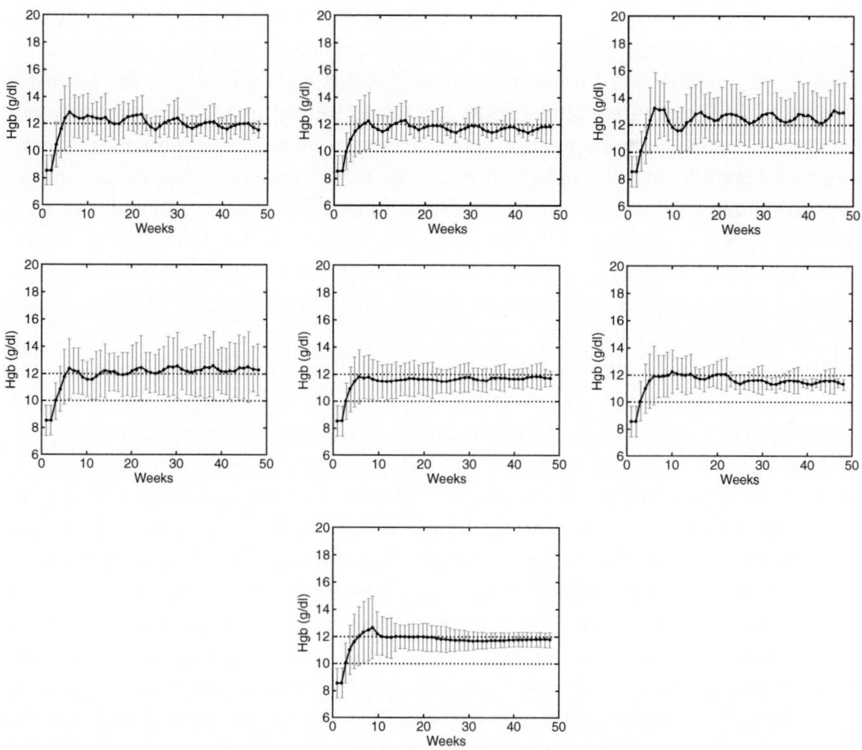

Fig. 18.1 Simulation of different paper anemia management protocols submitted for evaluation to The Renal Network 9 and 10. At the time, the hemoglobin target was 10–12 g/dL

Other problems in developing a successful anemia management protocol is that patients within the population have a variable response [9]. This means that techniques designed around a one size fits all philosophy will on average work well for those patients in the center of this population but will perform very poorly for those patients that either respond very well or very poorly to administered erythropoietin. This is evidenced in the phenomenon known as hemoglobin cycling observed for many patients. Typically, for a patient that has a low hemoglobin, erythropoietin doses are escalated even when there is a positive movement in hemoglobin concentration. Then, there is a failure to reduce erythropoietin dose once the hemoglobin concentration has moved into the target range and it is not until hemoglobin succeed 12 g/dL that a decision is made to either reduce or stop dosing. Because of the nature of the erythropoietin response and the need for erythropoietin to support the maturation of precursor cells, holding erythropoietin doses leads to loss of these precursor cells and accentuates the rapid fall in hemoglobin resulting in cycling. This pattern of erythropoietin dosing leads to an average number of dose changes in patients per year at about six with of range of 0–11 [10].

The result of erythropoietin dosing algorithms based on expert opinion is that the hemoglobin average for the population is driven by the identified target range and not by individual need. As shown in Fig. 18.1, these expert systems do not uniformly achieve hemoglobin's in the middle of the target range, rather achieved hemoglobin is variable. This is primarily due to the lack of testing of the algorithms prior to implementation to determine how patients will respond to the proposed algorithm. In these cases, adjustments are made following use in actual patients. Research shows that the population standard deviation of these approaches is in the range of 1.5 g/dL and this information can be used to predict what percent of the population can exist within a specific target range. For instance, in order to have 66% of the population in target the target range would need to have a range of 3 g/dL. The other consequences of dosing algorithms for erythropoietin based on an expert system is the need for multiple and frequent dose changes which results in hemoglobin cycling.

The use of other techniques to improve upon drug dosing of erythropoietin has incorporated the use of artificial neural networks [11, 12]. An artificial neural network is a mathematical representation of a biological neuron where we have a series of inputs similar to dendrites that are connected to a hidden layer that represents the body of the neuron and an output similar to the axon. These mathematical neurons are arranged in at least two layers and process information in a nonlinear fashion similar to logistic regression. This structure allows the flexibility to model any nonlinear process. Contextually the artificial neural network is thought to simulate associative reasoning and training of the network is an iterative process designed to minimize the error between the predicted and observed parameter of interest. This is done through a process of supervised learning where each case is presented with paired input information and the desired outcome. In our first instance of applying this technique to the prediction of future hematocrit and hematocrit standard deviation we used inputs of current and past hematocrit, current and past hematocrit

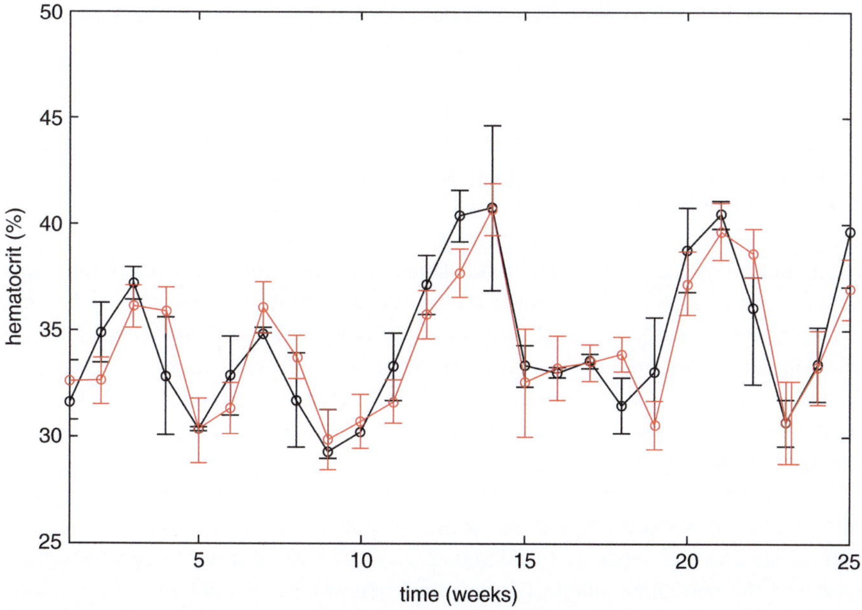

Fig. 18.2 Demonstration of the ability of the artificial neural network to predict hematocrit over time with the prediction in red and observed in black

standard deviation, and current and past erythropoietin dose. We predicted future hematocrit and hematocrit standard deviation [11]. Results of this prediction are shown in Fig. 18.2.

The construction of a model of hemoglobin response was the first step in the development of a decision support tool for anemia management. In pharmacokinetic terms this is the development of a pharmacodynamic model of erythropoietin response. The difference is that a pharmacodynamic model would be pre-defined and then its ability to predict would be tested by looking at data but with an artificial neural network the data is used to define the model.

One could then use this artificial neural network in a brute force approach and test the administration of every dose combination determining the hematocrit response and selecting the desired dose based on these combinations in an iterative fashion. However, a more sophisticated approach would be to incorporate control theory into the process and allow the artificial neural network to interact with a controller in a feedback loop to optimize treatment goals. One such approach is called model predictive control. Model predictive control is an advanced method of process control used in many aspects of engineering. It relies on a dynamic model of the process one is attempting to control which might be an artificial neural network. The model is used to predict the behavior of certain dependent variables such as hemoglobin and the input erythropoietin dose. The unique feature of feedback control that improves prediction is the way the controller accounts for errors in the prediction. When an error between observed and predicted occurs, the controller can make adjustments within its operating parameters to improve future predictions.

In the biological case of erythropoiesis, the kidney serves as the controller monitoring oxygen content in the blood on a second by second timeframe. The kidney then manipulates the production of erythropoietin in response to measured oxygen. The blood then delivers the erythropoietin to the bone marrow where it has is action on the creation of red blood cells which in turn enter the circulation and alter the oxygen-carrying capacity of the blood. This results in a feedback to the kidney in a new oxygen level which then can fine tune erythropoietin production. This process is interrupted in end-stage kidney disease where the kidneys ability to monitor oxygen content and produce erythropoietin may be compromised. In practice, we have replaced the second by second timeframe of monitoring oxygen content of the blood by the kidney with intermittent monitoring performed on a frequency usually of no greater than once a week.

A model predictive control technique was developed for the management of anemia of chronic kidney disease and tested in patients on hemodialysis [13]. The control structure consists of two separate computer programs one representing a model of the patient encoded as an artificial neural network and a dose optimizer. The artificial neural network has as its inputs the dose of erythropoietin and as its output a predicted hemoglobin. The dose optimizer is provided information on the target hemoglobin and the doses of erythropoietin available. The optimizer interrogates the patient model to determine the optimal dose of erythropoietin to achieve the target at a future date. In this case, that future date is 3 months from the current date. This delay is predicated on the fact that red blood cell lifespan in dialysis patients is compromised when compared to a patient with normal kidney function. Simulations using this approach resulted in less hemoglobin cycling then predicting 1 month ahead.

The development of the artificial neural network model of patients response to erythropoietin is a data requiring process. In this case, data from 186 dialysis patients comprised of combinations of erythropoietin dose and hemoglobin response are used two develop the artificial neural network. That model needs to be validated against a separate data set to ensure that the model generalizes appropriately. One limitation of an artificial neural network approach is that it will extrapolate poorly outside of the range of data used in training. This means that data that were generated when the hemoglobin target was 10–12 mg/dL may not be successfully used if the target range changes to a different range. When this change has the potential to occur one should incorporate a more physiologic model as we have done in our subsequent work [14].

A randomized controlled clinical trial of model predictive control in anemia management using an artificial neural network as the patient model was performed [15]. This study randomized 60 patients to either an active control group or treatment group using the model predictive controller. Following randomization subjects

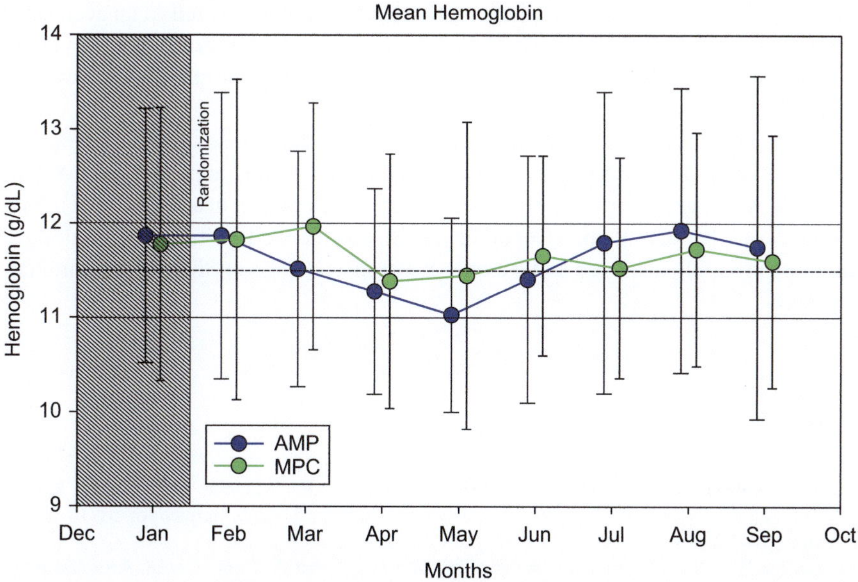

Fig. 18.3 Achieved hemoglobin following randomization to the anemia management protocol control group (AMP) and model predictive control group (MPC)

entered a 2-month washout period followed by 6 months for data collection. The target range for hemoglobin during the study was 11–12 g/dL in the prediction horizon for the model predictive controller was 3 months in the future. The results of that trial are shown in Fig. 18.3.

Use of the model predictive control algorithm resulted in the removal of hemoglobin cycling in the population and maintenance of those subjects randomized to model predictive control at or near the middle of the target range. Hemoglobin variance in those subjects in the model predictive control group was less than those in the anemia management protocol control group.

Following the successful completion of this randomized controlled clinical trial we performed a retrospective review of the anemia management protocol and model predictive control with a new target of 11.0 g/dL. In the anemia management protocol group hemoglobin's fell from 11.5 to 11.3 g/dL while in the model predictive control group hemoglobin fell to 11.1 g/dL. Erythropoietin dose fell in the anemia management protocol group from 10,777 to 8743 U/week and fell in the model predictive control group from 9029 to 5902 U/week.

Proof that this approach can be exported to a dialysis facility in which the product was developed and to a different form of erythropoietin stimulating agent was demonstrated in a facility in New York. This facility used darbepoetin as its erythropoietin stimulating agent. The facility was averaging doses of darbepoetin in the range of 80–100 μg per patient per week prior to implementation of the Smart anemia manager. Following implementation darbepoetin doses fell to an average of about 30 μg per patient per week. The percent of patients within the facilities target range of 9.5–11 g/dL initially fell from about 40 to 33% but quickly improved to greater than 45%.

This work on the use of artificial intelligence in the management of anemia of chronic kidney disease has demonstrated superiority of this approach over a standardized anemia management protocol. The approach results in a decrease in hemoglobin variability at both the level of the patient and the facility. Target hemoglobin's are more precisely achieved and patients are exposed to less erythropoietin stimulating agent.

References

1. Sealfon RSG, Mariani LH, Kretzler M, Troyanskaya OG. Machine learning, the kidney, and genotype-phenotype analysis. Kidney Int. 2020;97:1141–9. https://doi.org/10.1016/j.kint.2020.02.028.
2. Becker JU, Mayerich D, Padmanabhan M, Barratt J, Ernst A, Boor P, et al. Artificial intelligence and machine learning in nephropathology. Kidney Int. 2020;98:65–75. https://doi.org/10.1016/j.kint.2020.02.027.
3. Lemley KV. Machine learning comes to nephrology. J Am Soc Nephrol. 2019;30:1780–1. https://doi.org/10.1681/ASN.2019070664.
4. Zhang J, Friberg IM, Kift-Morgan A, Parekh G, Morgan MP, Liuzzi AR, et al. Machine-learning algorithms define pathogen-specific local immune fingerprints in peritoneal dialysis patients with bacterial infections. Kidney Int. 2017;92:179–91. https://doi.org/10.1016/j.kint.2017.01.017.
5. Akbilgic O, Obi Y, Potukuchi PK, Karabayir I, Nguyen DV, Soohoo M, et al. Machine learning to identify dialysis patients at high death risk. Kidney Int Rep. 2019;4:1219–29. https://doi.org/10.1016/j.ekir.2019.06.009.
6. Tomasev N, Glorot X, Rae JW, Zielinski M, Askham H, Saraiva A, et al. A clinically applicable approach to continuous prediction of future acute kidney injury. Nature. 2019;572:116–9. https://doi.org/10.1038/s41586-019-1390-1.
7. Degoulet P. Artificial intelligence—its use in nephrology. Nephrol Dial Transplant. 1987;2:298–303.
8. Bennett WM, Aronoff GR, Morrison G, Golper TA, Pulliam J, Wolfson M, et al. Drug prescribing in renal failure: dosing guidelines for adults. Am J Kidney Dis. 1983;3:155–93. https://doi.org/10.1016/s0272-6386(83)80060-2.
9. Lacson E Jr, Ofsthun N, Lazarus JM. Effect of variability in anemia management on hemoglobin outcomes in ESRD. Am J Kidney Dis. 2003;41:111–24. https://doi.org/10.1053/ajkd.2003.50030.
10. Fishbane S, Berns JS. Hemoglobin cycling in hemodialysis patients treated with recombinant human erythropoietin. Kidney Int. 2005;68:1337–43. https://doi.org/10.1111/j.1523-1755.2005.00532.x.
11. Gaweda AE, Muezzinoglu MK, Aronoff GR, Jacobs AA, Zurada JM, Brier ME. Individualization of pharmacological anemia management using reinforcement learning. Neural Networks. 2005;18:826–34. https://doi.org/10.1016/j.neunet.2005.06.020.
12. Gaweda AE, Muezzinoglu MK, Aronoff GR, Jacobs AA, Zurada JM, Brier ME. Using clinical information in goal-oriented learning. IEEE Eng Med Biol Mag. 2007;26:27–36.

13. Gaweda AE, Jacobs A, Aronoff GR, Brier ME. Model predictive control of erythropoietin administration in the anemia of ESRD. Am J Kidney Dis. 2008;51:71–9. https://doi.org/10.1053/j.ajkd.2007.10.003.
14. Gaweda AE, Aronoff GR, Jacobs AA, Rai SN, Brier ME. Individualized anemia management reduces hemoglobin variability in hemodialysis patients. J Am Soc Nephrol. 2014;25:159–66. https://doi.org/10.1681/ASN.2013010089.
15. Brier ME, Gaweda AE, Dailey A, Aronoff GR, Jacobs AA. Randomized trial of model predictive control for improved anemia management. Clin J Am Soc Nephrol. 2010;5:814–20. https://doi.org/10.2215/CJN.07181009.

Chapter 19
Pathogenesis of Coronary Artery Disease in Chronic Kidney Disease: Strategies to Identify and Target Specific Populations

Clinton Brown and Ernie Yap

Coronary Artery Disease in People with Chronic Kidney Disease

Coronary artery disease (CAD) increases in prevalence and severity as kidney function declines. Accelerated atherosclerosis and increased cardiovascular (CVD) events have been extensively documented in patients with chronic kidney disease (CKD) and end stage renal diseases (ESRD) [1, 2]. In the USA between 1980 and 2000, mortality from CVD disease in people with CKD remained substantially higher than the general population even as the overall CVD mortality fell by more than 40% within the same time period [3, 4]. This can be partially explained by the observation that ESRD patients have atypical presentation of myocardial injury due to the presence of exercise intolerance or diabetes. As well, they exhibit non-classical changes on electrocardiograms [5]. Diagnostic biomarkers such troponins are chronically elevated in ESRD patients and thus simple thresholds are unreliable; all of which leads to under-recognition and delays in treatment. Nevertheless, the phenomenon of "reverse epidemiology," that is; higher cholesterol, blood pressure, and BMI, have been reported to predict a better outcome in these individuals [6] suggests the presence of a distinct set of biological risk factors peculiar to the ESRD state. The correlation between inflammation in uremia and atherosclerotic disease was demonstrated by Stenvinkel et al. who reported an association between C-reactive proteins and carotid intima-media area among people with diminished renal function [7]. Gennip et al. studied markers of endothelial dysfunction (sVCAM-1, E-selectin, P-selectin, thrombomodulin, sICAM-1, sICAM-3) and low grade inflammation (hs-CRP, SAA, IL-6, IL-8, TNF-α) in people with CKD not on

C. Brown · E. Yap (✉)
SUNY Downstate Health Sciences University, Brooklyn, New York, USA
e-mail: Clinton.Brown@downstate.edu

S. J. Saggi, M. O. Salifu (eds.), *Technological Advances in Care of Patients with Kidney Diseases*, https://doi.org/10.1007/978-3-031-11942-2_19

dialysis and ESRD and found that both groups had significantly higher levels of serum biomarkers of endothelial dysfunction and low-grade inflammation than controls [8].

Dyslipidemia in ESRD

The natural history and treatment of dyslipidemia among people with ESRD is well documented. The Die Deutsche Diabetes and Dialysis Study (4D trial) enrolled 1255 hemodialysis patients with type 2 diabetes and demonstrated that lowering LDL cholesterol with atorvastatin (20 mg per day) did not produce statistically significant reductions in the composite primary end point of CVD death, nonfatal myocardial infarction, and stroke [9]. This was followed by an international, multicenter, randomized, double-blind prospective trial—A study to evaluate the Use of Rosuvastatin in subjects On Regular hemodialysis (AURORA) that involved 2776 ESRD patients on hemodialysis randomized to receive rosuvastatin, 10 mg daily, or placebo. Participants in the intervention arm had lower LDL cholesterol level but had no significant effect on the composite primary end point of death from CVD causes, nonfatal myocardial infarction, or nonfatal stroke compared to their placebo counterparts [10]. The study of heart and renal protection trial (SHARP) enrolled 9270 patients who were randomly assigned to simvastatin plus ezetimibe (4650 patients; 230 on dialysis) versus placebo (4620 patients; 246 on dialysis) showed that patients on dialysis also did not appear to have as significant risk reduction in the primary outcome compared to patients with CKD not on dialysis although the trial did not have sufficient power to assess these effects on dialysis and non-dialysis patients [11]. A subsequent meta-analysis of dialysis patients receiving statin therapy that include the 4D, AURORA, and SHARP trials did not come to a definitive conclusion on the utility of statin therapy, as results did not reach statistical significance even though CKD patients not on dialysis were found to have a statistically significant benefit [12].

Lipoprotein (a) is an independent risk factor for CVD [13] and is elevated in many individuals with CKD or ESRD and is especially elevated in individuals with CKD and proteinuria [14]. However, whether Lp(a) contributes to CVD risk in patients with CKD or ESRD has not been confirmed. Large randomized clinical trials are needed to assess the impact of Lp(a) on CVD in the CKD population.

Taken together, the above suggests that the routine lipid profile per se is not a predominant influence in predicting atherosclerotic CVD risk in people with ESRD. Although competing factors in conjunction with more advanced CKD contributing to CVD outcomes may dilute the effect of dyslipidemia in clinical trials, other factors peculiar to the uremic state such as p-cresyl sulfate, inflammatory cytokines [8, 15] or modified lipoproteins due to carbamylation, oxidation, and glycation [16]. Heretofore unknown mechanisms may also be involved.

Pathogenesis of CAD in CKD: New Insights

Endothelial dysfunction is characterized by impaired endothelium-dependent vasorelaxation and represents an early step in the pathogenesis of atherosclerosis [17]. It is principally driven by uremia induced generation of reactive oxygen species (ROS) that triggers production of advanced glycation end products (AGE); notably *N*ε-(carboxymethyl)lysine (CML) which in turn leads to a self-perpetuating positive feedback interconnecting cycles of oxidation and inflammation. In this metabolic setting ROS functions as the initiator while CML functions as a connecting factor (Fig. 19.1).

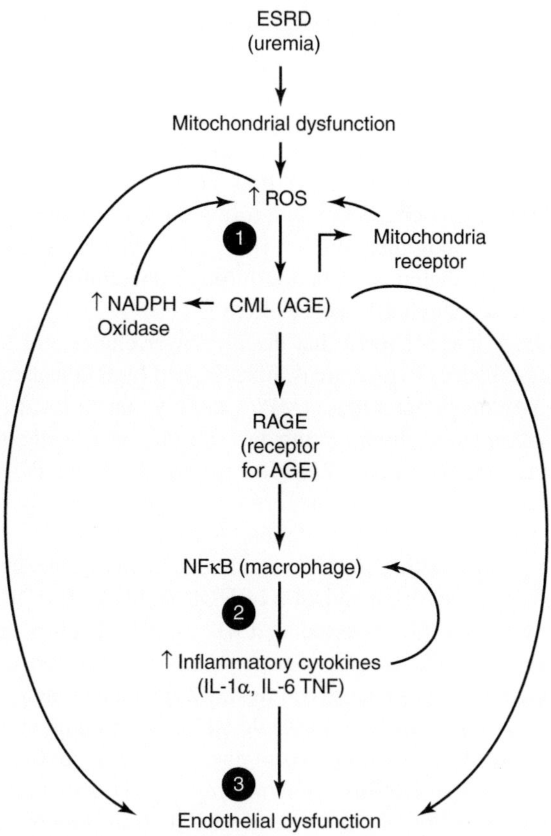

Fig. 19.1 Interconnecting positive feedback loops (cycles) of oxidation and inflammation induced by uremia in ESRD. (1) Uremia induced mitochondrial dysfunction causing elevated ROS (oxidation). ROS triggers production of CML (AGE). CML activates NADPH Oxidase and mitochondria receptor and both actions reciprocally triggers ROS generation (positive feedback). (2) CML binds to its receptor, RAGE, and activates the proinflammatory macrophage receptor NFκB releasing inflammatory cytokines (IL-1α, IL-6 TNF) which in turn feedback to reactivate NFκB (positive feedback). (3) Inflammatory cytokines, CML, and ROSs either individually or combine to cause endothelial dysfunction. *Legend*: *AGE* advanced glycation end products, *CML N*ε-(Carboxymethyl) lysine, *IL-1α* interleukin 1 alpha, *IL-6* interleukin-6, *NFκB* nuclear factor kappa B, *RAGE* receptor for advanced glycation end product, *ROS* reactive oxygen species, *TNF α* tumor necrosis factor alpha

CML escalates an inflammatory process by inducing macrophage activation and release of cytokines such as interleukin-1α, interleukin-6, and tumor necrosis factor [18]. Cytokines so generated can feedback and activate macrophage receptor (NFκB) resulting in further cytokine production. The key components of these interacting cycles, inflammatory cytokines, ROS, and AGE (CML) individually or combined, trigger, and exacerbate endothelial dysfunction.

Protein Carbamylation

The metabolic perturbations in the ESRD state predisposes to protein carbamylation, which is a form of irreversible posttranslational protein modification (PTPM) that occurs via adduction with isocyanic acid (a spontaneous dissociation product of urea) on either the N-terminus of proteins or free amino acids (Nα-carbamylation) or the Nε-amino group of protein lysine residues forming carbamyl-lysine (homocitrulline) [19]. Other forms of modified (lipo) proteins caused by the PTPM mechanism that promote atherosclerotic plaque formation are oxidation of LDL [20] and glycation (i.e., CML, and other AGEs) [16]. Carbamylated LDL has been demonstrated to induce endothelial dysfunction through uncoupling of endothelial nitric oxide (NO) synthase, which then acts as ROS [21].

In mice models, it was shown that despite lower cholesterol levels, mice with CKD had increased aortic plaque areas, fibrosis, and luminal narrowing in conjunction with increased myeloperoxidase (MPO) activity that co-localized with infiltrating lesional macrophages, highlighting the role of macrophage-derived MPO in CKD-accelerated atherosclerosis [22] Macrophage-derived MPO accelerates multiple phases of the atherosclerotic process by catalyzing oxidation of thiocyanate, which in turn causes protein carbamylation by cyanate [23].

However, in patients with ESRD, elevated ambient urea concentration appears to be the dominant driver of carbamylation of HDL and LDL (cHDL, cLDL). In uremic patients, cHDL elevation is associated with impaired antioxidant function [24, 25], decreased reverse cholesterol transport activity, impaired cholesterol efflux capacity [26], decreased endothelial cell repair [24], and increased foam cell formation [27]; the latter highlights a remarkable and ironic finding about carbamylated HDL, that is, its transformation into a pro-atherogenic lipoprotein.

In addition, cholesterol efflux from macrophage is also impaired in uremia-induced reduced expression of ABCA1 and ABCG1 transporters. This further complicates lipid efflux and potentiates lipid accumulation in macrophages which further contributes to foam cell transformation [28].

In the physiological state, pyrophosphate (PPi) plays an essential role in suppressing calcification. Protein carbamylation suppressed the expression of ectonucleotide pyrophosphate/phosphodiesterase 1, a key enzyme in the generation of pyrophosphate, thereby decreasing the supply of PPi resulting in ectopic vascular medial calcification [29]. Consequently, in the ESRD state, there is a high risk of enhanced CV burden due calcification of the atherosclerotic plaque and vascular media.

Macrophage Function in ESRD

CD36 belongs to the class B scavenger receptor family, which also includes scavenger receptor B1 and lysosomal integral membrane protein 2 and is encoded by *CD36* gene, located on chromosome 7 (7q11.2) and consists of 15 exons. Its extensive glycosylation is required for intracellular trafficking onto the cell membrane. In patients with ESRD, monocytes/macrophages upregulate scavenger expression CD36 thus increasing its efficiency in removing lipoproteins that have been modified as a consequence of urea toxicity; resulting in an increased influx of modified lipoproteins in arterial wall macrophages [30]. Macrophage CD36 interacts with oxidized LDL, which triggers signaling cascades for inflammatory responses that recruit immune cells (monocytes) into the intima wall leading to their eventual morphological transformation into foam cells; an early critical stage of atherosclerosis [31].

Autophagy

Autophagy is a cellular process of lysosome-mediated degradation of cytoplasmic components or damaged organelles in response to cellular stress [32]. Although it primarily serves a protective role to maintain cellular homeostasis and ensure cell survival, it can also play a role in cell death [33]. Autophagy occurs at low basal levels in virtually all cells and is rapidly up regulated during high demand states, such as starvation and ischemia [32, 34, 35]. Autophagy plays a key role in removing defective organelles such as mitochondria a process that prevents oxidative stress, cellular dysfunction and apoptosis [36, 37].

Autophagy is impaired in ESRD, leading to incomplete lysosomal degradation of autophagosome content resulting in accumulation of ROS, auto-phagolysosomes endosomes, and lipid droplets, and their decreased efflux [38]. Impaired autophagy especially effects survival of terminally differentiated cells like kidney podocytes and cardiomyocytes [39–41].

To this point, in 2015, a clinical trial involving people with type 2 diabetes with impaired glomerular filtration rate (GFR) when treated with the sodium-glucose cotransporter 2 (SGLT2) inhibitor empagliflozin, demonstrated significantly lower rates of death from CVD causes [42] and this finding was subsequently replicated in other SGLT2 inhibitors [43]. These agents inhibit the SGLT2 glucose transporter found in the S1 segment of the proximal tubule which is responsible for 90% of glucose reabsorption in the kidney, resulting in glucosuria and improving the glycemic index. They also ameliorate glomerular hyperfiltration, exerting additional hemodynamic benefits. The CREDENCE trial compared canagliflozin against placebo in more than 4000 people with type 2 diabetes already on renin-angiotensin-aldosterone (RAAS) inhibition and showed lower risk of CVD death in the SGLT2-inhibitor cohort [44].

These positive signals on CVD outcomes provoked speculation regarding the mechanism of action of SGLT2 inhibitors beyond that of its salutary effects on renal hemodynamics [45]. For example, these agents have shown consistent effects in increasing hematocrit by augmenting erythropoietin production due to its hypoxia ameliorating effects on neural crest-derived fibroblasts in the early proximal tubule [46]. Concomitantly, as it transmits tubular workload distally to the S3 segment of the proximal tubule and medullary thick ascending limb, the relative hypoxia there stimulates the release of hypoxia-inducing factors (HIF), promulgating enhanced erythropoietin production [47]. Intriguingly, SGLT2 inhibitors also reduce levels of inflammatory markers that characterize the chronic inflammation state implicated in atherogenesis, such as NFκB, interleukin-6, monocyte chemoattractant protein 1, fibronectin, matrix metalloproteinase-7 [48–50].

SIRT1 is a NAD^+-dependent deacetylase that modulates the generation of endothelial NO, a protective factor for promoting endothelium-dependent vascular relaxation by activating endothelial NO synthase [51], which promulgates an anti-atherosclerotic effect. However, SIRT 1 also acts as a principal sensor of glucose depletion. In patients with CKD not on dialysis, SGLT2 inhibitors create a starvation state by continuous off-loading glucose into the urine and thereby stimulating the activity of SIRT1 [52] which in turn activates autophagy. Preservation of autophagy restores mitochondria generation, and this may explain the favorable outcomes in renal and cardiac functions in diabetic patients with CKD on SGLT2 inhibitors as demonstrated in recent clinical trials [42–44].

In summary, in ESRD, increased CD36 expression on macrophages, dysregulated autophagy and uremia-induced PTPM (especially of lipoproteins) synergistically cohere to promulgate an arterial obstructive syndrome; independent of traditional risk factors of coronary artery disease [53].

Strategies to Identify and Target Specific Populations

The risk of CVD events including death is strikingly increased with higher stages of CKD. On the basis of several meta-analyses of clinical trial data, statin therapy is recommended by the National Lipid association (NLA) and the Kidney Disease: Improving Global Outcomes guidelines (KDIGO) for patients with CKD not on dialysis [54, 55]. However, in patients with ESRD, therapies that target pivotal steps along inflammatory, lipid/lipoprotein, and glycation pathways, to date have been disappointing [9–11, 56].

There have been novel approaches in treating statin-resistant dyslipidemia. Proprotein convertase subtilisin kexin 9 (PCSK9) is a serine protease that catalyzes degradation of hepatocyte LDL receptors and thus, increased LDL cholesterol. PCSK9 inhibitors have been shown to be safe and effective in lowering LDL levels and other atherogenic lipid fractions [including lipoprotein (a)], myocardial infarctions and all-cause mortality [57, 58], their usage in people with ESRD has been reported to be safe and efficacious [59] but has not yet been evaluated in a randomized clinical trial. The promising potential of SGLT2 inhibitors in mitigating CV morbidity and mortality in patients with CKD not on dialysis [44] requires further study beyond their anti-glycemic potential.

Over the years, the only therapeutic modality that has been shown to significantly improve CVD mortality in patients with ESRD on hemodialysis has been the restoration of renal function with a successfully transplanted kidney [1, 2].

Future Directions

Innovations in diagnosing and treating CVD in CAD and ESRD remain an unmet medical need. Mechanistic pathways of uremia on lipoprotein modification, autophagy and lysosomal dysfunction, and inflammation, in contributing to atherosclerosis needs to be clarified. The use of novel biomarkers should be investigated. As well, the safety and efficacy of disease-modifying therapies at the primary and secondary prevention levels such as PCKS9 and SGLT 1 inhibitors should be rigorously pursued.

References

1. Sarnak MJ, Levey AS, Schoolwerth AC, et al. Kidney disease as a risk factor for development of cardiovascular disease: a statement from the American Heart Association Councils on kidney in cardiovascular disease, high blood pressure research, clinical cardiology, and epidemiology and prevention. Hypertension. 2003;42(5):1050–65. https://doi.org/10.1161/01.HYP.0000102971.85504.7c.
2. Foley RN, Parfrey PS, Sarnak MJ. Epidemiology of cardiovascular disease in chronic renal disease. J Am Soc Nephrol. 1998;9(12 Suppl):S16–23.
3. Ford ES, Ajani UA, Croft JB, et al. Explaining the decrease in U.S. deaths from coronary disease, 1980–2000. N Engl J Med. 2007;356(23):2388–98. https://doi.org/10.1056/NEJMsa053935.
4. Collins AJ, Kasiske B, Herzog C, et al. Excerpts from the United States renal data system 2006 annual data report. Am J Kidney Dis. 2007;49(1 Suppl 1):A6–7, s1–296. https://doi.org/10.1053/j.ajkd.2006.11.019.
5. Herzog CA, Littrell K, Arko C, Frederick PD, Blaney M. Clinical characteristics of dialysis patients with acute myocardial infarction in the United States: a collaborative project of the United States Renal Data System and the National Registry of myocardial infarction. Circulation. 2007;116(13):1465–72. https://doi.org/10.1161/circulationaha.107.696765.

6. Kalantar-Zadeh K, Block G, Horwich T, Fonarow GC. Reverse epidemiology of conventional cardiovascular risk factors in patients with chronic heart failure. J Am Coll Cardiol. 2004;43(8):1439–44. https://doi.org/10.1016/j.jacc.2003.11.039.
7. Stenvinkel P, Heimbürger O, Paultre F, et al. Strong association between malnutrition, inflammation, and atherosclerosis in chronic renal failure. Kidney Int. 1999;55(5):1899–911. https://doi.org/10.1046/j.1523-1755.1999.00422.x.
8. van Gennip ACE, Broers NJH, Ter Meulen KJ, et al. Endothelial dysfunction and low-grade inflammation in the transition to renal replacement therapy. PLoS One. 2019;14(9):e0222547. https://doi.org/10.1371/journal.pone.0222547.
9. Wanner C, Krane V, März W, et al. Atorvastatin in patients with type 2 diabetes mellitus undergoing hemodialysis. N Engl J Med. 2005;353(3):238–48. https://doi.org/10.1056/NEJMoa043545.
10. Fellström BC, Jardine AG, Schmieder RE, et al. Rosuvastatin and cardiovascular events in patients undergoing hemodialysis. N Engl J Med. 2009;360(14):1395–407. https://doi.org/10.1056/NEJMoa0810177.
11. Baigent C, Landray MJ, Reith C, et al. The effects of lowering LDL cholesterol with simvastatin plus ezetimibe in patients with chronic kidney disease (study of heart and renal protection): a randomised placebo-controlled trial. Lancet. 2011;377(9784):2181–92. https://doi.org/10.1016/S0140-6736(11)60739-3.
12. Upadhyay A, Earley A, Lamont JL, Haynes S, Wanner C, Balk EM. Lipid-lowering therapy in persons with chronic kidney disease: a systematic review and meta-analysis. Ann Intern Med. 2012;157(4):251–62. https://doi.org/10.7326/0003-4819-157-4-201208210-00005.
13. Nordestgaard BG, Langsted A. Lipoprotein (a) as a cause of cardiovascular disease: insights from epidemiology, genetics, and biology. J Lipid Res. 2016;57(11):1953–75. https://doi.org/10.1194/jlr.R071233.
14. Wanner C, Rader D, Bartens W, et al. Elevated plasma lipoprotein(a) in patients with the nephrotic syndrome. Ann Intern Med. 1993;119(4):263–9. https://doi.org/10.7326/0003-4819-119-4-199308150-00002.
15. Jing YJ, Ni JW, Ding FH, et al. p-Cresyl sulfate is associated with carotid arteriosclerosis in hemodialysis patients and promotes atherogenesis in apoE−/− mice. Kidney Int. 2016;89(2):439–49. https://doi.org/10.1038/ki.2015.287.
16. Bucala R, Makita Z, Vega G, et al. Modification of low density lipoprotein by advanced glycation end products contributes to the dyslipidemia of diabetes and renal insufficiency. Proc Natl Acad Sci U S A. 1994;91(20):9441–5. https://doi.org/10.1073/pnas.91.20.9441.
17. Gimbrone MA Jr, García-Cardeña G. Endothelial cell dysfunction and the pathobiology of atherosclerosis. Circ Res. 2016;118(4):620–36. https://doi.org/10.1161/circresaha.115.306301.
18. Rectenwald JE, Moldawer LL, Huber TS, Seeger JM, Ozaki CK. Direct evidence for cytokine involvement in neointimal hyperplasia. Circulation. 2000;102(14):1697–702. https://doi.org/10.1161/01.cir.102.14.1697.
19. Stark GR, Stein WH, Moore S. Reactions of the cyanate present in aqueous urea with amino acids and proteins. J Biol Chem. 1960;235(11):3177–81. https://doi.org/10.1016/S0021-9258(20)81332-5.
20. Diepeveen SH, Verhoeven GH, van der Palen J, et al. Oxidative stress in patients with end-stage renal disease prior to the start of renal replacement therapy. Nephron Clin Pract. 2004;98(1):c3–7. https://doi.org/10.1159/000079921.
21. Speer T, Owala FO, Holy EW, et al. Carbamylated low-density lipoprotein induces endothelial dysfunction. Eur Heart J. 2014;35(43):3021–32. https://doi.org/10.1093/eurheartj/ehu111.
22. Zeng L, Mathew AV, Byun J, Atkins KB, Brosius FC 3rd, Pennathur S. Myeloperoxidase-derived oxidants damage artery wall proteins in an animal model of chronic kidney disease-accelerated atherosclerosis. J Biol Chem. 2018;293(19):7238–49. https://doi.org/10.1074/jbc.RA117.000559.
23. Wang Z, Nicholls SJ, Rodriguez ER, et al. Protein carbamylation links inflammation, smoking, uremia and atherogenesis. Nat Med. 2007;13(10):1176–84. https://doi.org/10.1038/nm1637.

24. Sun JT, Yang K, Lu L, et al. Increased carbamylation level of HDL in end-stage renal disease: carbamylated-HDL attenuated endothelial cell function. Am J Physiol Renal Physiol. 2016;310(6):F511–7. https://doi.org/10.1152/ajprenal.00508.2015.
25. Holzer M, Zangger K, El-Gamal D, et al. Myeloperoxidase-derived chlorinating species induce protein carbamylation through decomposition of thiocyanate and urea: novel pathways generating dysfunctional high-density lipoprotein. Antioxid Redox Signal. 2012;17(8):1043–52. https://doi.org/10.1089/ars.2011.4403.
26. Anderson JLC, Gautier T, Nijstad N, et al. High density lipoprotein (HDL) particles from end-stage renal disease patients are defective in promoting reverse cholesterol transport. Sci Rep. 2017;7:41481. https://doi.org/10.1038/srep41481.
27. Holzer M, Gauster M, Pfeifer T, et al. Protein carbamylation renders high-density lipoprotein dysfunctional. Antioxid Redox Signal. 2011;14(12):2337–46. https://doi.org/10.1089/ars.2010.3640.
28. Cardinal H, Raymond M-A, Hébert M-J, Madore F. Uraemic plasma decreases the expression of ABCA1, ABCG1 and cell-cycle genes in human coronary arterial endothelial cells. Nephrol Dial Transplant. 2006;22(2):409–16. https://doi.org/10.1093/ndt/gfl619.
29. Mori D, Matsui I, Shimomura A, et al. Protein carbamylation exacerbates vascular calcification. Kidney Int. 2018;94(1):72–90. https://doi.org/10.1016/j.kint.2018.01.033.
30. Chmielewski M, Bryl E, Marzec L, Aleksandrowicz E, Witkowski JM, Rutkowski B. Expression of scavenger receptor CD36 in chronic renal failure patients. Artif Organs. 2005;29(8):608–14. https://doi.org/10.1111/j.1525-1594.2005.29097.x.
31. Jiang Y, Wang M, Huang K, et al. Oxidized low-density lipoprotein induces secretion of interleukin-1β by macrophages via reactive oxygen species-dependent NLRP3 inflammasome activation. Biochem Biophys Res Commun. 2012;425(2):121–6. https://doi.org/10.1016/j.bbrc.2012.07.011.
32. Takeshige K, Baba M, Tsuboi S, Noda T, Ohsumi Y. Autophagy in yeast demonstrated with proteinase-deficient mutants and conditions for its induction. J Cell Biol. 1992;119(2):301–11. https://doi.org/10.1083/jcb.119.2.301.
33. Mizushima N, Levine B, Cuervo AM, Klionsky DJ. Autophagy fights disease through cellular self-digestion. Nature. 2008;451(7182):1069–75. https://doi.org/10.1038/nature06639.
34. Yorimitsu T, Klionsky DJ. Autophagy: molecular machinery for self-eating. Cell Death Differ. 2005;12 Suppl 2(Suppl 2):1542–52. https://doi.org/10.1038/sj.cdd.4401765.
35. Zhang J, Ney PA. Role of BNIP3 and NIX in cell death, autophagy, and mitophagy. Cell Death Differ. 2009;16(7):939–46. https://doi.org/10.1038/cdd.2009.16.
36. Glick D, Barth S, Macleod KF. Autophagy: cellular and molecular mechanisms. J Pathol. 2010;221(1):3–12. https://doi.org/10.1002/path.2697.
37. Kim I, Rodriguez-Enriquez S, Lemasters JJ. Selective degradation of mitochondria by mitophagy. Arch Biochem Biophys. 2007;462(2):245–53. https://doi.org/10.1016/j.abb.2007.03.034.
38. Lin TA, Wu VC, Wang CY. Autophagy in chronic kidney diseases. Cells. 2019;8:1. https://doi.org/10.3390/cells8010061.
39. Hartleben B, Gödel M, Meyer-Schwesinger C, et al. Autophagy influences glomerular disease susceptibility and maintains podocyte homeostasis in aging mice. J Clin Invest. 2010;120(4):1084–96. https://doi.org/10.1172/jci39492.
40. Fang L, Li X, Luo Y, He W, Dai C, Yang J. Autophagy inhibition induces podocyte apoptosis by activating the pro-apoptotic pathway of endoplasmic reticulum stress. Exp Cell Res. 2014;322(2):290–301. https://doi.org/10.1016/j.yexcr.2014.01.001.
41. Maejima Y, Isobe M, Sadoshima J. Regulation of autophagy by Beclin 1 in the heart. J Mol Cell Cardiol. 2016;95:19–25. https://doi.org/10.1016/j.yjmcc.2015.10.032.
42. Zinman B, Wanner C, Lachin JM, et al. Empagliflozin, cardiovascular outcomes, and mortality in type 2 diabetes. N Engl J Med. 2015;373(22):2117–28. https://doi.org/10.1056/NEJMoa1504720.

43. Kosiborod MN, Jhund PS, Docherty KF, et al. Effects of Dapagliflozin on symptoms, function, and quality of life in patients with heart failure and reduced ejection fraction. Circulation. 2020;141(2):90–9. https://doi.org/10.1161/CIRCULATIONAHA.119.044138.
44. Perkovic V, Jardine MJ, Neal B, et al. Canagliflozin and renal outcomes in type 2 diabetes and nephropathy. N Engl J Med. 2019;380(24):2295–306. https://doi.org/10.1056/NEJMoa1811744.
45. Esterline RL, Vaag A, Oscarsson J, Vora J. Mechanisms in endocrinology: SGLT2 inhibitors: clinical benefits by restoration of normal diurnal metabolism? Eur J Endocrinol. 2018;178(4):R113–r125. https://doi.org/10.1530/eje-17-0832.
46. Sano M, Goto S. Possible mechanism of hematocrit elevation by sodium glucose cotransporter 2 inhibitors and associated beneficial renal and cardiovascular effects. Circulation. 2019;139(17):1985–7. https://doi.org/10.1161/CIRCULATIONAHA.118.038881.
47. Mazer CD, Hare GMT, Connelly PW, et al. Effect of Empagliflozin on erythropoietin levels, iron stores, and red blood cell morphology in patients with type 2 diabetes mellitus and coronary artery disease. Circulation. 2020;141(8):704–7. https://doi.org/10.1161/circulationaha.119.044235.
48. Heerspink HJL, Perco P, Mulder S, et al. Canagliflozin reduces inflammation and fibrosis biomarkers: a potential mechanism of action for beneficial effects of SGLT2 inhibitors in diabetic kidney disease. Diabetologia. 2019;62(7):1154–66. https://doi.org/10.1007/s00125-019-4859-4.
49. Dekkers CCJ, Petrykiv S, Laverman GD, Cherney DZ, Gansevoort RT, Heerspink HJL. Effects of the SGLT-2 inhibitor dapagliflozin on glomerular and tubular injury markers. Diabetes Obes Metab. 2018;20(8):1988–93. https://doi.org/10.1111/dom.13301.
50. Han JH, Oh TJ, Lee G, et al. The beneficial effects of empagliflozin, an SGLT2 inhibitor, on atherosclerosis in ApoE (−/−) mice fed a western diet. Diabetologia. 2017;60(2):364–76. https://doi.org/10.1007/s00125-016-4158-2.
51. Mattagajasingh I, Kim CS, Naqvi A, et al. SIRT1 promotes endothelium-dependent vascular relaxation by activating endothelial nitric oxide synthase. Proc Natl Acad Sci U S A. 2007;104(37):14855–60. https://doi.org/10.1073/pnas.0704329104.
52. Ying Y, Jiang C, Zhang M, Jin J, Ge S, Wang X. Phloretin protects against cardiac damage and remodeling via restoring SIRT1 and anti-inflammatory effects in the streptozotocin-induced diabetic mouse model. Aging (Albany NY). 2019;11(9):2822–35. https://doi.org/10.18632/aging.101954.
53. Falk E, Shah PK, Fuster V. Coronary plaque disruption. Circulation. 1995;92(3):657–71. https://doi.org/10.1161/01.cir.92.3.657.
54. Jacobson TA, Ito MK, Maki KC, et al. National lipid association recommendations for patient-centered management of dyslipidemia: part 1—full report. J Clin Lipidol. 2015;9(2):129–69. https://doi.org/10.1016/j.jacl.2015.02.003.
55. Wanner C, Tonelli M. KDIGO clinical practice guideline for lipid management in CKD: summary of recommendation statements and clinical approach to the patient. Kidney Int. 2014;85(6):1303–9. https://doi.org/10.1038/ki.2014.31.
56. Freedman BI, Wuerth JP, Cartwright K, et al. Design and baseline characteristics for the aminoguanidine clinical trial in overt type 2 diabetic nephropathy (ACTION II). Control Clin Trials. 1999;20(5):493–510. https://doi.org/10.1016/s0197-2456(99)00024-0.
57. Navarese EP, Kołodziejczak M, Schulze V, et al. Effects of proprotein convertase Subtilisin/Kexin type 9 antibodies in adults with hypercholesterolemia. Ann Intern Med. 2015;163(1):40–51. https://doi.org/10.7326/M14-2957.
58. Sabatine MS, Giugliano RP, Keech AC, et al. Evolocumab and clinical outcomes in patients with cardiovascular disease. N Engl J Med. 2017;376(18):1713–22. https://doi.org/10.1056/NEJMoa1615664.
59. González Sanchidrián S, Labrador Gómez PJ, Aguilar Aguilar JC, Davin Carrero E, Gallego Domínguez S, Gómez-Martino Arroyo JR. Evolocumab for the treatment of heterozygous familial hypercholesterolemia in end-stage chronic kidney disease and dialysis. Nefrologia. 2019;39(2):218–20. https://doi.org/10.1016/j.nefro.2018.09.005.

Index

S. J. Saggi, M. O. Salifu (eds.), *Technological Advances in Care of Patients with Kidney Diseases*, https://doi.org/10.1007/978-3-031-11942-2